PHYSICAL ACTIVITY AND H
HONG KONG YOUT

Physical Activity and Health of Hong Kong Youth

EDITED BY

David P. Johns

AND

Koenraad J. Lindner

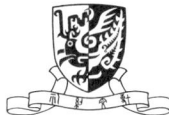

The Chinese University Press

Physical Activity and Health of Hong Kong Youth
   Edited by David P. Johns and Koenraad J. Lindner

© **The Chinese University of Hong Kong**, 2006

ISBN 962–996–238–1

THE CHINESE UNIVERSITY PRESS
The Chinese University of Hong Kong
SHA TIN, N.T., HONG KONG
Fax: +852 2603 6692
    +852 2603 7355
E-mail: cup@cuhk.edu.hk
Web-site: www.chineseupress.com

Printed in Hong Kong

Table of Contents

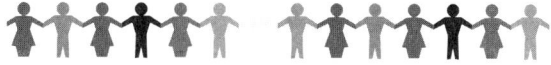

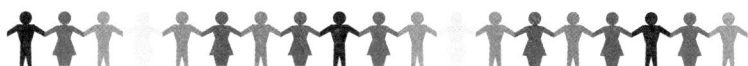

CHAPTER 1

Introduction

David P. Johns

Physical activity has attracted the interest of various agencies whose primary interest is the promotion of health. Numerous studies have demonstrated that there is an inverse dose-response relationship between physical activity and various chronic diseases (Hardman & Stensel 2003). In addition, physical activity seems to have a positive effect on an individual's psychological and emotional well being. Although most studies have been conducted in developed societies, the results indicate that regardless of ethnicity, culture and geography, physical activity may be a common component of health. The purpose of this book is not only to make a statement about the health status of a particular group in a particular region, but to show also that evidence found in a particular culture provides the validity for research constructs and processes that are assumed to be universal.

By using accepted methods of investigation employed in other countries throughout the world, the research reported and the recommendations made in this book assume common grounds from which comparative analyses can be made. As Hong Kong is a burgeoning city whose population is expected to increase dramatically over the next decade, it represents a standard by which other cities throughout the world can judge the extent to which the future health and well-being of its citizens are threatened. The statement that emerges from this book reflects a view of health that is at once universal and distinctive. First, the statement may be unique because health behaviours are examined against the distinct and unique cultural and psychological background of a Chinese society. Second, the statement reflects the common concern that the Hong Kong community shares with the global community over the future health of the population by paying particular attention to the state of its youth.

The focus on the young people of Hong Kong rather than the general population has been chosen for two reasons. First, there is compelling evidence to suggest that the burden of ill health in adults can be attributed to their lifestyles when they were young (Armstrong, McManus, Welsman, & Kirby 1996; Hardman 2001; Hardman & Stensel 2003) and that the roots of disease are found in the socialized behaviours of childhood making it necessary to discover what determines the levels of physical activity in children and any risks that such levels may present. Second, there is a lack of research on children's health-related physical activity, and "relatively little evidence [that] unambiguously relates childhood physical activity or fitness to childhood health, a more favourable childhood risk profile, or to later adult health." (Boreham & Riddoch 2001, 916–917) Nevertheless, it has been suggested that habitual physical activity among youth populations should be promoted (American Academy of Pediatrics 2000) to prevent the loss of adult functional capacity and reduce the risk of their premature morbidity and mortality. Therefore, much more work is required to clarify the role that physical activity plays in the lives of children in order to describe the impact of urban living on the health of children in large cities such as Hong Kong.

The Region

The environments in which societies develop do not simply influence their members but they also reflect their desired way of life. This is clearly observed particularly in densely populated urban areas such as Hong Kong where the built environment reflects the aspirations of its citizens but at the same time shapes their lives in terms of where they live, work, enjoy their leisure and how they travel. The environment is therefore a profound but complex influence on the lifestyle of the individual and is often taken for granted until it becomes dysfunctional or threatens the way of life or the health of its citizens. It is against the background of this densely populated urban region that the research is reported and the discussions are presented in this book.

The rise of the modern city is usually but not always associated with a rise in industrial development (Giddens 1997). Most cities in developing countries have increased their capacity to accommodate rising populations but the infrastructure that sustains a reasonable standard of living has not kept pace. Hong Kong is a typical modern urban centre that has been transformed from a manufacturing economy to one that has embraced information and services. Hong Kong comprises not only a city, but also a region "of islands, a peninsula, its hinterland and land reclaimed from the sea" (Sweeting 1998, 7), and is a Special Administrative Region of the People's Republic of China that was once a colony of Britain. The rise of the city to international status reflected the post-World War II economic development that transformed a small British trading port into a major international financial and trading centre in the world by 1993 (Sweeting 1998). The Special Administrative Region of Southern China, in which Hong Kong is located, was set up as an administrative measure under the "One Country Two Systems" policy to facilitate the repatriation of the territory back to China in 1997. The city, strategically placed at the edge of the Pearl River Delta, was established in 1842 as a free port and as a secure base for trade with China. Everyday life of the mono-cultural population of almost 7 million is shaped by deep cultural values and beliefs, but is subject to a "whole range of exogenous forces" (Sweeting 1998, 9) that has imposed non-Chinese influences on the economic, political and cultural development that are disproportionate to the population being served. These forces were the result of an occupation by a colonial power that has recently given way to an alternative force being exerted by the People's Republic of China. It is these forces that have indirectly attracted many of the contributors of this book to examine the cultural, social and environmental influences on the health and physical activity patterns of Hong Kong youth. Adopting Western models of analysis, they have been sensitive to the particular cultural values and beliefs, and in doing so they have tested the universal assumptions that are often attached to such models. By examining the physical activity and the health of youth in a Chinese culture, they have not only clarified "the tension between distinctiveness and commonality" (Bond 1996, xix) but have also demonstrated that similarities found among societies are not discounted because of specific differences.

Theoretical Underpinnings and Contributions

Attempting to explain why some people are active while others are not, has become a very challenging task (Sallis and Owen 1999). Nevertheless, to understand the variety of forces that influence and effect health-related behaviours is important because it may lead to information that will assist in effective intervention. Since the influences that affect human behaviours are complex and diverse, no single model or theory provides a complete or even thorough understanding of what determines active and sedentary lifestyles. Early psychological theories were thought to contain the answers but they have given way to health belief models that were later characterized by broader theories such as the social cognitive theory of Bandura (1986). Bandura's ideas have been shown to be relevant and sufficiently encompassing to accommodate the complexity of human behaviour. More recently efforts to understand physical activity have been developed by means of an ecological model proposed by Sallis and Owen (1999). This model is the logical extension of Bandura's theory but encompasses a multiple-level approach to uncovering the determinants of physical activity by examining social systems, public policies and physical environments that are found in the setting being examined. This model is useful in examining the influence that a robust market economy may have on the traditions of Chinese society, but it obviously cannot claim to assist in the analysis of the biological research reported in some of the chapters to follow.

Although this model may well apply to the many studies and their authors' perspectives that are included in this book, an even more recent model known as the "social determinants of health and environmental health promotion" (Northridge, Sclar, & Biswas 2004, 557) has emerged that would also be useful in attempting to understand the relationship between health and built environments.

In Hong Kong, the high density of urban life including inadequate design of buildings, vehicular traffic, erosion, deterioration, pollution, intensive use of energy, subhuman living conditions and the lack of child space impact on the amount of physical activity and its relationship to health. Although the model does not refer directly to physical activity and will not be used in this volume, Northridge, Sclar and Biswas have proposed a conceptual framework that should not be overlooked in an effort to understand the broader implications of built environments.

The New Public Health

We think it is true to say that this book aligns with what Petersen and Lupton (1996) called the "New Public Health" in which the concern over the health of the society has turned from the control of filth, odour and contagion generated when the growth of 19th century cities outpaced progress in urban design, to focusing on the social and personal factors of risk that have arisen from changing lifestyles (Petersen & Lupton 1996). Lifestyle has been transformed into a manageable risk factor that is believed to lead to the control of what have become known as "lifestyle diseases" and in particular cardiovascular disease (Gard & Wright 2001). This new perspective on health coincides with how modern societies are characterized by global environmental concerns, the potential hazards that modern societies face and how these are managed by the degree of risk to which modern urban life exposes its citizens (Beck 1992a; 1992b).

Currently, a biomedical discourse that typifies the response to risk has identified lifestyle as the variable upon which our attention must be focused. In particular, physical activity is singled out as the one behaviour that "has beneficial effects on most (if not all) organ systems and consequently it helps to prevent a broad range of health problems and diseases" (U.S. Department of Health and Human Services 2002, 9). Physical activity in this context is defined as "any bodily movement produced by contraction of skeletal muscles that substantially increase energy expenditure" (Kesaniemi et al. 2001, S351). How much physical activity (or in medical terms the 'dose') is needed to obtain a health benefit is described in terms of the frequency, duration, intensity and type of activity that is accomplished during work or discretionary time. The product of these terms yields a total energy expenditure that relates to the ability to perform physical activity and is defined in terms of endurance and strength known as physical fitness. Therefore, physical activity and health, rather than physical fitness, have become the focus of attention for researchers wishing to understand more about the dose-response relationship and how it can be applied to the reduction of risk of chronic disease. Sedentary behaviours are therefore regarded as risk factors in an age when inactive lifestyles seem to be more prevalent than in any period in history.

Risk is now recognized in terms of hazards against which there is no insurance; only the hope that exposure to risk can be reduced (Gard & Wright 2001). In the US, the "Behavioural Risk Factor Surveillance System" (U.S. Department of Health and Human Services 2002) informs the public of the appearance of diseases such as diabetes and obesity and to what extent they are reaching epidemic proportions. In the UK, a report from the Chief Medical Officer provides the current evidence of the impact of physical activity on health which indicates that "people who are physically active reduce their risk of developing major chronic diseases" (Department of Health 2004 iii). This relatively recent emphasis on monitoring the risks of a society is one of the characteristics of the new public health that has brought with it a proliferation of new sub-disciplines. Out of the many health-related professions that have emerged, biomedical researchers in health-related physical activity, attempt to establish a relationship between physical activity and health that they believe "should be the cornerstone of contemporary public health" (Bouchard 2001).

Unfortunately, this relationship is more difficult to understand than was first thought. There is substantial evidence to suggest that adequate physical activity results in a reduction in chronic diseases and if we would encourage urban societies to be less sedentary, the reduction in risk could become a reality. Based on this premise, the solution seems to be a simple one, yet the precise formulation of the type and volume of activity that is necessary to reduce risk continues to baffle exercise scientists. Precisely how much more activity is required to offset the risk of disease is currently being debated among researchers but no exact prescription has yet been provided (Bouchard

2001). The only agreement that has been reached among the experts is that physical activity should be promoted among the young. But consensus clearly does not ensure implementation as energy expenditures continue to decline.

Other Considerations

The debate over dose-response issues has now extended to school physical education where some have suggested that major gains in changing a society from sedentary to active can be made (Sallis & McKenzie 1991). Unfortunately, the acceptance of a biomedical model in school physical education as visualized by Sallis and McKenzie (1991) does not take place in spite of their convincing arguments. This failure is due to several forces that have not been taken into account, not the least of which is a lack of evidence upon which claims of certainty are made. Moreover, the biomedical model seems to have overlooked the fact that human activity is a category of behaviour that is not independent of race, age, gender and practically all social and cultural influences. There may also be a danger in valorizing a model that promotes solutions as "remarkably simple in appearance" (Bouchard and Blair, quoted in Gard and Wright 2001, 547) and dismisses the complexity and plurality of the issues surrounding health promotion.

There are other dangers that have emerged in the valorization of physical activity as the way to better health. A technology has emerged in which certain behaviours are favoured over others and a sense of personal responsibility has been constituted. Even though the emphasis now changes from physical fitness to physical activity, there is a tendency to prescribe how one should live by considering disease as either "an individual property or an external threat" (Petersen & Lupton 1996, 174) to which one must assume moral responsibility through an active lifestyle. It is not surprising that students do not embrace a physical education programme that ostensibly focuses on physical activity as a method of alleviating chronic disease by creating binary oppositions that normalize certain alternatives as morally wrong. A number of opposing binaries come to mind, such as fit and unfit, "good performance and bad performance, normal and abnormal, active and passive. This kind of reductionism, based on a dose and response formula, is far too restrictive considering the "plurality of difference that exists in the social world" (Lupton 1995, 159) and it tends to increase rather than reduce anxiety among the population.

Exercise scientists suggest that the physical education curriculum could be re-contextualized in order to emphasize health (Gard & Wright 2001). The underlying assumption is that by increasing the amount of activity during physical education, children's health risks will be reduced. If the solution to the problem of inactivity was as simple as this claim suggests, then all children would eventually change their lifestyle habits to include more physical activity and thereby increase energy expenditure and solve the problem. However, this is not the case as the habits of the younger generation continue to be a cause for concern among health workers. Such a simplistic solution overlooks the way in which power structures work on and through the body (Lupton 1995). For example, school physical education has recently been deemed an ideal site because it is situated in the only institution that is able to "address health-related physical activity needs of virtually all children" (Sallis & McKenzie 1991, 124). However, when students in modern urban schools are encouraged to pursue an active lifestyle, it is necessary to take into consideration that they are also vulnerable to consumer markets forces. These forces are far more powerful and convincing than a school curriculum that continues to offer traditional games and sports as a means by which disease and ill health are prevented. We have to take into account that youths in their resistance to the dictums of everyday life are more willing and, in fact, able to derive greater pleasure and satisfaction from alternative youth cultural practices that tend to be the antithesis of the purpose of exercise and physical activity. Schools adopting the re-contextualized model will be more likely to succeed if they can work with consumer cultures rather than against them. It seems that the consumer media culture is to be understood as a niche market that is associated with the symbolic production, experiences and practices that are part of the symbiotic development of "post-industrialization, the advertising industry and the image media" (Kenway & Bullen 2001, 11). The present generation of young people is far too sophisticated as a special group of consumers to be told what is good for them.

In order to reduce the danger of drawing conclusions that may lead to the belief that changing lifestyles can be easily accomplished, we want to ensure that those who read this book become aware of the difficulties facing workers in health-related fields in changing the behaviours of the urban populations. In order to focus on these difficulties, the chapters in this book are drawn from a wide range of perspectives including medicine, education, health and sports science. While these disciplines are often regarded as unrelated to each other, researchers from these disciplines, for the purpose of this book, have been brought together in a common cause. The thread that runs through all their work is that they are engaged in various forms of practice and research that inform them that health is at risk when physical activity is trivialized, ignored or discouraged. Diversification of backgrounds serves the need for a multi-disciplinary approach in order to better understand the complexity of a modern urban life and how these complexities deserve serious consideration if future health is to be improved. The backgrounds include professionally trained individuals who are engaged in teaching at universities in a range of subjects. Some are clinicians, medical practitioners and/or researchers working in hospitals and research centres while others are exercise scientists who teach and research in university departments.

The Synopsis

The fourteen chapters of this book are arranged in five parts to accommodate the various approaches that have been taken to understand the relationship between physical activity and the health of young people. Part one comprises two chapters on the assessment of physical fitness and physical activity. In Chapter 1, Stephen Wong describes the nature of physical activity and how it is operationalized and evaluated as a research variable. In Stanley Hui's chapter that follows, specific issues that have surrounded the measurement and evaluation of fitness in children are introduced. He describes a study that employs a revised fitness testing protocol that has recently been utilized to establish fitness norms for Hong Kong children. These norms will be useful for all those who read this book and for those who are particularly interested in using the norms for comparisons.

The second part of the book provides evidence of the extent to

which Hong Kong children and youth are active. In Chapter 3, Duncan
Macfarlane reports three studies which consistently show that Hong
Kong children do not compare well with other countries in terms of
the frequency and levels of intensity of physical activity. He
demonstrates that the amounts of activity in which Hong Kong children
and youth participate fall short of international standards
recommended for the development and maintenance of good health.
The next chapter, by Alison McManus, examines physical activity as a
behavioural and biological complexity. While most of our research
examines the behavioural aspects of children's physical activity, the
biological function is often overlooked. This oversight masks the
importance of physical activity as the mechanism that promotes both
motor and neural development. If we continue to examine present
sedentary populations as normal populations, we may fail to make the
connection between biology and behavourism. This section concludes
with a chapter by Cindy Sit, Ken Chow and Koenraad Lindner that
documents further evidence that young people in Hong Kong are
generally active, examines motives for the engagement in physical
activities and analyses factors influencing physical activity participation.

The third part of the book is devoted to the examination of a
research conducted in hospital settings indicating that early symptoms
of chronic diseases of adulthood now appear in children. A particularly
troubling problem for health workers is the increasing prevalence of
child obesity in Hong Kong. In Chapter 6, Rita Sung and Tony Nelson
show that obesity may have its early beginnings in the sedentary
lifestyles of children. They are led to the conclusion that although it is
difficult to directly link physical activity with obesity, physical activity
may nevertheless be an important component in the fight to reduce
obesity. In Chapter 7, Neil Thomas, Norman Chan, Clive Cockram
and Brian Tomlinson provide a detailed justification for the concerns
that health workers have raised about the health impact that overweight
and obesity have on cardiovascular risk factors. Because the
relationship between these conditions is intricate and treatment
limited, the best policy at the present time is to attempt to reduce or
prevent child obesity. One of the promising and least expensive way
to reduce such health complications would be to encourage young
people to be more active.

Part four of the book examines the influencing factors that have been observed in the behaviours of Hong Kong Youth and how these various environmental, social and psychological factors consciously and unconsciously influence the choices that we make in terms of their participation in physical activity. In Chapter 8, Cecilia Au presents the findings of her study on Hong Kong youth and the influence of socializing agents that are thought to influence participation patterns and rates. One of her findings is that peer influence such as that from friends and the school physical education teacher is the strongest socializing force for Hong Kong youth, rather than the family. In Chapter 9, David Johns examines education policy, implementation and school practice to illustrate how institutional factors influence young people's participation. In the final chapter in Part Four, David Johns and Patricia Vertinsky examine how the physical environment coupled with the social structure combines to form an ecology that influences families and youth in their choice of physical activity.

The chapters in Part Five have been written to show what must be considered to reduce the sedentary inclination of a modern developed societies such as Hong Kong. In Chapter 11, Jim Dickinson writes from a community medical perspective and makes a connection between physical inactivity and the health outcomes. Although he promotes the preventative role of medicine, he also suggests a community-wide approach to improving the urban environment in order that opportunities for physical activity may assume a rightful place in the lifestyles of urban dwellers. In Chapter 12, Amy Ha and Graham Fishburne provide a pragmatic approach by first highlighting the health concerns associated with physical inactivity. Then they describe some of the health intervention studies which attempt to increase the physical activity by a new curriculum that has recently been proposed to encourage educational change in Hong Kong. Finally, they strongly suggest that our focus must be turned to promoting physical education by targeting young people and competing with the commercial industries that promote the logos of popular culture. In the closing chapter, Koenraad Lindner presents his views on the implications of the facts and concepts as presented in this book on the future of school physical education in Hong Kong.

References

American Academy of Pediatrics 2000. Physical fitness and activity in schools. *Pediatrics* 105:1156–1157.

Armstrong, N., McManus, A., Welsman, J. & Kirby, B. 1996. Physical activity patterns and aerobic fitness among prebubescents. *European Physical Education Review* 2: 19–29.

Bandura, A. 1986. *Social foundations of thought and action: A social cognitive theory.* Englewood Cliffs, NJ: Prentice Hall.

Beck, U. 1992a. *Risk society.* London: Sage.

———. 1992b. From industrial society to risk society: Questions of survival, social structure and ecological enlightenment. *Theory, Culture and Society*: 9:97–123.

Bond, M. H. 1996. *The handbook of Chinese psychology.* Hong Kong: Oxford University Press.

Boreham, C. and C. Riddoch 2001. The physical activity, fitness and health of children. *Journal of Sports Sciences* 19:915–929.

Bouchard, C. 2001. Physical activity and health: Introduction to the dose-response symposium. *Medicine and Science in Sports and Exercise* 3:S347–S350.

Gard, M., and J. Wright 2001. Managing uncertainty: Obesity discourses and physical education in a risk society. *Studies in Philosophy and Education* 20: 535–549.

Giddens, A. 1997. *Sociology.* London: Polity Press.

Hardman, A. 2001. Physical activity and health: Current issues and research needs. *International Journal of Epidemiology* 30: 1193–1197.

Hardman, A. E. and D. J. Stensel 2003. *Physical activity and health: The evidence explained.* London, UK: Routledge.

Kenway, J., & E. Bullen 2001. *Consuming children: Education — education — aadvertising.* Buckingham, UK: Open University Press.

Kesaniemi, Y. A., E. Danforth, and M. D. Jensen, P. G. Kopelman, P. Lefebvre and B.R. Reeder 2001. Dose-response issues concerning physical activity and health: An evidence-based symposium. *Medicine & Science in Sports & Exercise* 33, 6:S351–S358.

Lupton, D. 1995. *The imperative of health: Public health and the regulated body.* London, UK: Sage Publications.

Northridge, M. E., E. D. Sclar and P. Biswas 2004. Sorting out the connections between the built environment and health: A conceptual framework for navigating pathways and planning health cities. *Journal Urban Health* 80,4: 556–568.

Petersen, A. and D. Lupton 1996. *The new public health: Health and self in the age of risk.* London, UK: Sage Publications.

Sallis, J. and T. MacKenzie 1991. Physical education's role in public health. *Research Quarterly for Exercise and Sport* 62:124–137.

——— and N. Owen 1999. *Physical activity & behavioural medicine.* London, UK: Sage Publications.

Sweeting, A. 1998. Education and development in Hong Kong. In P. Stimpson & P. Morris, eds. *Curriculum and assessment for Hong Kong.* Hong Kong: Open University Press, 5–50.

U.S. Department of Health and Human Services 2002. *Physical activity fundamental to preventing disease.* Washington D.C.: Office of the Assistant Secretary for Planning and Evaluation.

PART I

Methodological Issues in Physical Activity Research

The first section of this book comprises two chapters dealing with measurement matters. The chapter by Wong and Sum examines techniques for the assessment of energy expenditure. Three groups of methods are discussed, namely, subjective measures (such as self-reports), secondary measures (such as heart rate monitoring), and criterion measures (such as calorimetry). The authors explain the techniques, discuss their pros and cons and cite validity and reliability estimates from the literature. The reader obtains a good appreciation of the intricacies of physical activity measurement.

In Chapter 3, Stanley Hui takes the assessment of physical fitness as his topic. He explains the importance of measuring fitness and presents an historical overview of fitness testing philosophy and methodology. A comparison of existing fitness test batteries allows insight into the strengths and weakness of various approaches. Hui presents a rationale for and the protocol of the CUHK Test for Health-Related Fitness along with a reprint of the Hong Kong norm tables compiled from this test for males and females between the age 9 to 19.

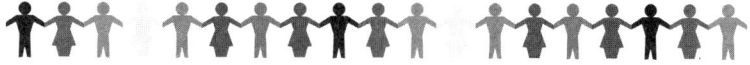

CHAPTER 2

Physical Activity in Children: the Measurement Issues

Stephen H. S. Wong and Raymond K. W. Sum

Introduction

Current data indicate that the prevalence of individuals who are either overweight or obese is increasing in both adult and child populations throughout the world (WHO 2002). Studies have shown that obesity is associated with less favorable cardiovascular and metabolic risk factor profiles in children (Daniels, Morrison, Sprecher, Khoury, & Kimball, 1999; Lauer and Clarke, 1989; Sung, Tong, Yu, Lau, Mok, Yam, et al., 2003). However, although the etiology of obesity is still unclear, physical inactivity has been identified as possibly one of the controllable risk factors (Booth, Chakravarthy, Gordon, & Spangenburg, 2002). There are several reasons that may explain the prevalence of sedentary lifestyles among children in developed countries and regions. These explanations have predominantly social, environmental and psychological characteristics.

Physical activity (PA) has been suggested as a possible solution and is defined as the amount of work performed (watts) or it can be expressed as time period of activities (hrs) or units of movement (counts). It is usually measured in three dimensions: duration, frequency, intensity (strenuousness) and in units such as kcal/min, KJ/hr (Montoye, Kemper, Saris, & Washburn, 1996). Alternatively, it is defined as any bodily movement produced by the contraction of the skeletal muscle that increases energy expenditure above the baseline level (Wuest & Bucher, 2003; Sirard & Pate, 2001). In particular, low PA levels have been associated directly with TV viewing, playing video games and inversely with time engaged in PA outdoors (Gortmaker, Must, Sobol, Peterson, Colditz, & Dietz, 1996; Janz, Levy, Burns, Torner, Willing, Warren, 2002; Robinson, 1999). Dietary intake is also an important factor in obesity. In the present generation there is evidence to suggest a tendency among Hong Kong children towards eating foods that are higher in fat and sugar, reflecting similar trends in other developed countries (Fu & Hao, 2002; Leung, Lee, Lui, Ng, Peng & Luo, 2000). They are also more likely to spend a large part of their free time in sedentary activity such as watching television or playing computer games. Understanding the PA levels in young children may be particularly critical in the prevention of adult obesity since the age at which body fat reaches a post-infancy low point (typically 4–6 years) is inversely associated with obesity later in life. However, in spite of the sophisticated technical equipment now available, an accurate assessment of PA in children and adolescents continues to be a challenge.

The purpose of this chapter is to review the current understanding and practice of the techniques in use for the assessment of energy expenditure in children and adolescents. The review will also provide a general overview of existing validation studies.

Human Energy Expenditure and Assessment Methods

Clearly, energy expenditure (EE) is related to body size. A small but active person may still expend fewer calories in 24 hr than a comparatively larger person who lives a sedentary lifestyle. In the human body, energy can be expended in three ways: The first is by maintaining resting metabolic activities (RMR), i.e., involuntary muscle activities account for 60–65% of thermogenic energy expenditure (TEE). The second is through non-exercise activity induced thermogenesis (NEAT) or dietary induced thermogenesis, also called thermic effect of food, the energy required for digestion. The third type of EE is through skeletal muscle activities or physical activities. Examples of this are maintaining posture, exercise, etc. which is the most variable factor (30–100% of BMR) among population. In order to assess the EE of PA among children and adolescents, at least six categories of techniques have been used. These include self-report, electronic or mechanical monitoring, direct observation, indirect calorimetry, doubly labeled water, and direct calorimetry. Each technique has inherent strengths and weaknesses. These will be discussed in subsequent sections of this chapter. Undoubtedly, the methods of assessing PA among elderly, adults, young children, and adolescents are necessarily different. Based on the purpose of the assessment, the techniques of estimating PA will be adjusted accordingly. Careful selection of the particular technique to be used is therefore crucial for a study. The diagram below summarizes the validation scheme of various methods, with the acceptable criterion measures indicated by arrows.

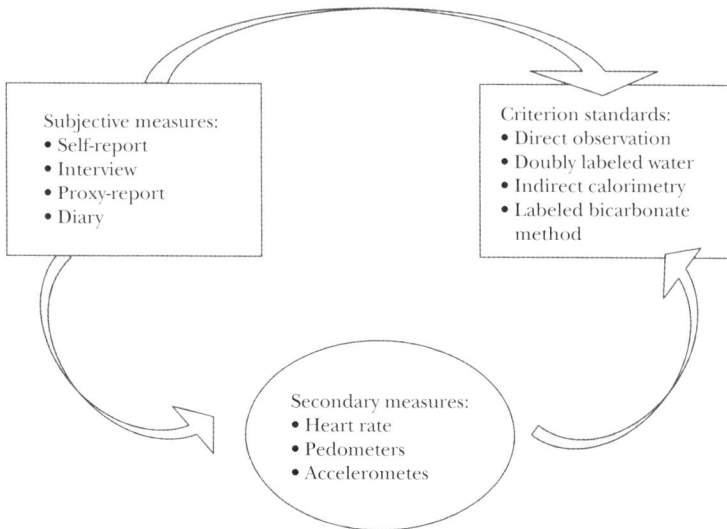

Direct observation is a more practical and comprehensive criterion measure for physical activity research. Secondary measures provide objective assessment of physical activities. Validating one of these measures against other secondary measures provide little insight into the instruments' true validity (Grund, Dilbe, Forberger, Krause, Siewers, Rieckert, et al., 2000; Sirard, Melanson, & Li, 2000).

Application, Advantage, Characteristic and Limitations of Each Assessment

Self-Report Measures

Many studies have used questionnaires to estimate children's PA. The measures can be classified into four major types, namely self-administered questionnaires, interviewer-administered questionnaires, proxy-reports and diaries. Due to the difference in purpose and targeted information, there is a question of validity and a need for standardization of the questionnaires.

Validity and repeatability: An accurate questionnaire is both reliable and valid. Sallis, Strikmiller, & Harsha (1996) reviewed twenty-two studies of the validity and repeatability of different types of children's PA measures. In his review, the dimensions of assessment were compared. These included the mode, frequency, intensity, and the duration of PA, the time period and weekday/weekend covered, primary summary variables and items, respondent/staff burden, and time required, of different measures. Reliabilities of nine reports of self-administered measures were high for children ranging in age from 8–17 years. Six studies of interviewer-administered measures were acceptable, with younger children having lower reliabilities. Both direct (objective measure of PA) and indirect (using a criterion variable believed related to PA) validity data from the studies of interviewer-administered measures supported these measures. Validity data of those self-administered measures were limited. The validity data of PA diaries from two studies showed that self-record PA were highly associated with both direct and indirect validity criteria (Aadahl & Jorgensen, 2003; Sirard, Melanson, & Li, 2000). In addition, there were moderately strong associations between the activity monitor and reports from teachers. Sallis suggested that investigators should select the most appropriate measures to fulfill their study's objectives, and to test for the validity and reliability of the newly developed instruments. He also recommended that objective measures such as direct observation and activity monitors should be used for assessing physical activity in children younger than age 10.

The validity and reliabilities of PA measures have also been reviewed (Sirard & Pate, 2001). For the 11 studies of self-administered questionnaires, the reliability of those measures was acceptable, with the reliability coefficients ranged from 0.51 to 0.98. While there was a wide range ($r = -0.10$ to 0.88) of correlation coefficients between those measures and direct observation, heart rate, or motion detection, the range of coefficients may be attributed to the different instruments and criterion measures used. Regarding the 7 studies of interviewer-administered questionnaires, there was still a wide range of correlation for those measures, with less complex measures providing greater correlations. This could indicate that older children are more able to complete those types of measures. Only 4 studies of proxy-reports of children's PA were reviewed and thus limited information of reliability and validity were recorded. In addition, there were only a few studies that used the diary method for assessing children's PA. Of these, Sirard and Pate (2001) have suggested that based on the high level of participation required to maintain an activity diary, this type of measure has limited use especially in a pediatric population of children under the age of 10.

There are various types of questionnaires that are available for measuring PA. The following is a summary of some of the advantages and limitations of these measures.

Self-administered questionnaire: This type is to be completed by the children by reporting their activities on a preprinted form. It is the most common method used to assess physical activity in children because of its low cost, lack of staff requirement and relatively efficient administration time. This type of measurement has the ability to gather activity information over a period of time and to test large numbers of children in a short time (Crocker, Bailey, Faulkner, Kowalski, & McGrath, 1997). However, some children may have difficulty in recalling a wide range of variations in levels of daily activity for periods of up to a week.

Interviewer-administered questionnaire: Measurement of this type is usually administered to a number of subjects by trained interviewers in a set time interval over a period of time. This technique may improve a child's cognition and accuracy, but the presence of the interviewer may introduce additional reactive bias.

Proxy-report: This type of report consists of the teachers and parent ratings of children's activities and can avoid recall errors caused by children's cognitive limitations. However, the characteristics and perceptions of the proxy respondent may introduce additional sources of bias.

Diary: A popular form of data collection has been achieved by means of a diary that is completed by the children and involved coding PA throughout the day in a diary form. Since it is a task that requires a high level of participation, younger children may have difficulty in maintaining an activity diary. Adolescents may be able to complete the diary but the accuracy must be carefully considered. A well-structured format and the use of activity records could aid recall in children (Trost, Ward, McGraw, & Pate, 1999).

Calorimetry

The basis of calorimetry is that energy can neither be destroyed nor created but only interconverted between different forms. The amount of food consumed should equal the energy expended, provided that the stored energy in the individual remains constant.

Direct calorimetry: Direct calorimetry measures the heat that has been lost from the human body to the environment. It is usually a whole body measurement made with the confines of a sealed, insulated chamber or a heat exchange body suit. Heat production, O_2 consumption and CO_2 production are recorded. Non-evaporative heat in the form of radiation, convection, and conduction is lost; in addition to the heat is also lost through the evaporation of water. The method is based on thermodynamic laws and the fact that energy of food is converted to heat in the human body. The non-evaporative components of heat exchange are measured passively in terms of the temperature gradient across the walls of a poorly insulated chamber (gradient layer calorimetry) or actively by measuring the rate at which heat must be extracted from a chamber to avoid heat loss through well-insulated walls (heat sink calorimetry) Since evaporative heat loss affects the moisture content of the environment, an independent measurement is required (Murgatroyd, Shetty, & Prentice, 1993).

The heat loss of the subject is measured at rest or during exercise classically in an insulated room calorimeter. Typically, this is an insulated chamber made with thin rigid material (eg. Glass-reinforced epoxy resin). A temperature-sensing layer covering over the inner and outer wall surface directly measures heat. This layer is usually made of etching copper films bounded to each side of the wall material. The rate of change in the heat content of the calorimeter must be considerably less than the heat flux from the subject, in order to ensure the only heat flux is from the subject. This is generally achieved by controlling the outside temperature of the wall using a water jacket maintained at $\pm 0.001°C/min$. Re-circulating air to the water-cooled heat exchanger allows the measurement of temperature. Alternatively, the water flows across the heat exchanger. This is achieved by the ratio of temperature rise, heat produced by an electrical heater of known power input is calculated.

All heat entering or leaving the chamber, for example hot food, chilled or warm drinks, etc., should be noted by knowing the weight, temperature and specific heat capacity. Electrical heat sources such as electrical heater, light or television are to be kept outside the chamber to prevent the heat that is dissipated being recorded by a wattmeter.

The advantage of this whole-body direct calorimetry is that it responds rapidly and produces accurate, precise results. It also provides a stable environment for strictly controlled studies of other physiological activities. For example, whole-body direct calorimetry can be used in conjunction with the use of various forms of exercise, such as treadmill running or ergometer cycling. However due to the difficulty of combining other invasive measurements, this technique is confined to the creation and maintenance of a strictly artificial environment in order to achieve an accurate measurement. However, from a metabolic point of view, this method is not able to provide information on substrates metabolism for energy provision.

Indirect calorimetry: Indirect calorimetry is a technique that measures the rate at which heat is produced in the body, by the rates of respiratory gas exchange, O_2 consumption and CO_2 production. Heat measures are calculated on the basis of O_2 consumed during the energy metabolism within the body. Indirect calorimetry can be performed easily in children by using standard commercial equipment as performed in adults (Goran, 1998). There are no special assumptions or theoretical considerations in children. However, there may be important considerations for measurement conditions before and during the measurement of metabolic rate to achieve the need for having subjects lie still and quiet for 30 minutes. For example, basal metabolic rate is often understood to encompass measurements performed after a 10- to 12-hour fast in a non-aroused state, with minimal muscular movement. These conditions are often met in adults when measurements can be performed immediately on awakening after the subject has slept in the laboratory or clinical research center (Berke, Gardner, Goran, & Poehlman, 1992). This approach is viable and reproducible in young children (Figueroa-Colon, Franklin, Goran, Lee,, & Weinsier, 1996) but may not always be possible among adults.

One of the limitations of using indirect calorimetry to measure the resting metabolic rate is that measurements can be performed over only a very short time (usually 30 minutes). Measurements over 24 hours can be achieved by having subjects live in a metabolic chamber. An additional advantage of this approach is that activity and food intake can be monitored and controlled. The disadvantage is that the chamber environment is not habitual, especially because movement and PA may be restricted. In addition, the high cost of the artificial environment provided by such a chamber may discourage use in some studies. This is a sophisticated unit that requires large - scale engineering and the use of a non-portable gas analysis equipment. Consequently, this method is impractical for validating a survey that measures 'usual' or for measuring weekly physical activities. However it has been used effectively for validating heart rate monitors, pedometers, and accelerometers in laboratory settings (Sirard et al., 2001).

Doubly Labeled Water Method

The doubly labeled water (DLW) method is a noninvasive, unobtrusive method for measuring EE. The subjects are allowed to carry out daily activities freely during the investigation period, which typically lasts 7–14 days or longer and only the urine is collected and analyzed. It is now viewed as the gold standard for measuring EE.

Application of DLW: For this technique, subjects are required to ingest water that is enriched with oxygen isotope (O_2-18 or ^{18}O) and a hydrogen isotope deuterium (^2H). The isotopes are naturally occurring and are non-radioactive. The human body is capable of metabolizing O_2-18 as part of water ($H_2^{18}O$) and carbon dioxide ($C^{18}O_2$) whereas deuterium is excreted as part of water (^2H_2O), after 5–14 days of ingestion. The difference between the two rates of elimination is used to determine carbon dioxide output and hence EE (Montoye et al., 1996, Sirard et al., 2001)

Validation of DLW: The DLW technique has been validated against indirect calorimetry in adults (Schoeller & Webb, 1984) and infants (Jones, Winthrop, Schoeller, Swyer, Smith, Filler, & Heim, 1987). In Schoeller's study, results indicated that EE from the DLW method averaged 6% more than those from respiratory gas exchange with an 8% coefficient of variation. The latter study showed that there was no significant difference between EE by DLW and the amounts measured by the respiratory gas exchange method. The rate of carbon dioxide production calculated by DLW differed from corresponding RGE value by –0.9 ±6.2%. Jones et al. (1987) concluded that the DLW method is valid for determining EE even among infants.

Advantages and disadvantages: Despite the utility of the method, the relatively high expense and accessibility of the isotopes discourages its application in large-scale studies. In addition, accurate dietary records must be obtained during the measurement period for the EE measurement. Measurement must be taken over a three-day period and only TEE can be obtained. For this reason, information cannot be provided on specific days, specific activities, or for a day-to-day variability, energy expenditure and the thermic effect of a meal.

The major advantages of the DLW Method, however, are that (i) the technique is noninvasive and unobtrusive; (ii) measurements are performed under free-living conditions over extended periods (from 3 to 14 days); and (iii) the technique can be used to estimate activity EE when combined with measurement of resting metabolic rate.

Precision and errors: The DLW method is generally considered to be more accurate than any other method for measuring energy expenditure. Investigators have examined the DLW technique and suggested that it has a theoretical precision with an error rate of only 3% to 5% (Schoeller and Taylor, 1987). The experimental variability improved to ±8% under more controlled sedentary living conditions, which is closer to theoretical estimates (Goran, Poehlman, & Danforth, 1994). Based on its accuracy and reasonable precision, the DLW technique has been used as a standard measure of energy expenditure in humans (Goran, Hunter, & Nagy, 1997).

Labeled Bicarbonate Method

This technique involves the use of the isotope method to quantify the rate of CO_2 production and ultimately the energy cost of leisure activities. To determine the validity of this technique for measuring energy costs of leisure activity. Horswill, Zipf, & Kien (1997) compared values using isotope dilution with those obtained using indirect calorimetry during activities with varying energy costs: Eight adolescents were measured in the following activities watching television, playing a string instrument, and walking. Their results showed that CO_2 production by these two methods were comparable.

Heart Rate Monitoring

One technique that has been examined rigorously in children is the heart rate (HR) method (Yu, Sung, So, Lam, Nelson, Li, Yuan, & Lam, 2002). Some of the limitations of this technique are that it is time consuming, that it requires close cooperation from the subjects, and that there is some concern that HR may vary independently of EE. However, Armstrong (1998) exercised 98 children and adolescents aged 5 to 16 years old at different speeds on a treadmill. The data confirmed that regardless of age, brisk walking and jogging elicited steady-state HR of about 140 and 160 beats/min respectively. Consequently, HR data have been analyzed at thresholds of >=140 and >=160 beats/min to represent moderate PA (equivalent to brisk walking) and vigorous PA(equivalent to jogging) respectively.

The use of HR to estimate EE is based on the linear relationship between HR and O_2 consumption. The recorded HR values were converted to oxygen consumption (VO_2) and subsequently into EE, with the use of the established individual HR-VO_2 calibration curve. However, the relationship is not robust at the low end of PA spectrum.

To eliminate other factors that infer these results, such as psychological and environmental stress, FLEX HR technique has been used to limit these effects (Grund et al., 2000, Sirard et al., 2001).

The flex value for HR represents the HR unique to each person that distinguishes rest from exercise. During the period when HR falls below the flex value, EE is assumed to be equivalent to resting EE. In the entire group, total EE was estimated to be within 6–20% from HR data when compared with DLW, and the correlation between the two techniques was 0.91. (Livingstone, Coward, & Prentice, 1992).

Advantages and limitations: When compared to other measures, the HR monitoring method has the advantage of being objective in nature and not dependent on subject compliance. The HR monitor device consists of a transmitter, which is snapped into a cloth-tape chest electrode, and a lightweight receiver is worn at the subject's waist. The transmitter detects heart signals and sends electrical impulses to the circuitry of the pulse monitor. It is small and inexpensive and has the added advantage of being able to provide information on the intensity, duration and frequency of the activities. Subjects only need to wear the HR transmitter and the wrist receiver during the monitoring period. They do not have to wear them when bathing and sleeping. Each HR interval is timed and the pulse beats are averaged on a rolling basis. Data is updated every 5 minutes and recorded in memory every 60 seconds. Data recorded can be retrieved through an interface unit to a computer. The energy expenditure and the PA level can then be calculated from the heart rate. Although this is an efficient method of obtaining data, the main limitation is that HR can be influenced by other factors including emotional stress and body positioning during activity.

Motion Sensor

Based on the definition that PA is bodily movement producing EE, the motion senor method detects body movement that is then used to estimate physical activity. Various instruments are available for detection and are discussed in the following section.

Pedometers: These instruments detect the number of steps or mileage walked by the subject. Some models also calculate distance and estimate energy expenditure. It is used to record activities taking place in a vertical direction, and by means of its spring mechanism. Most commercially available pedometers are worn at the waist and are sensitive to vertical movement. The response will therefore be affected by position, mode of pedometer attachment, and movement style and walking speed of the individual being monitored. The activity pattern of children usually is characterized by brief bursts of moderate or high intensity physical activity in combination with periods of low intensity activity. However, the pedometer tends to have lower sensitivity for recording low intensity activities. (Kilanowski, Angela, & Leonard, 1999). Due to the variation that exists among models in regard to the internal mechanism and sensitivity, not all pedometers count steps accurately (Crouter, Schneider, Karabulut & Bassett, 2003; Schneider, Crouter, Lukajic, & Bassett, 2003; Schneider, Crouter & Bassett, 2004; Le Masurier, Lee & Tudor-Locke, 2004). Thus, it is important for researchers who use pedometers to assess PA to be aware of their accuracy and reliability (Melanson, Knoll, Bell, Donahoo, Hill, Nysse, Lanningham-Foster, Peters & Levine, 2004; Cyarto, Myers & Tudor-Locke, 2004).

Accelerometers: The first generation of this type of motor senor was the Caltrac. This model was a single plane accelerometer that accumulates counts or kilocalories over time. Newer motor sensors include the ActiGraph and the Tritrac accelerometers. Both of these models contain a memory that permits storage of data, where user can specify time intervals, such as counts per minutes, and allow quantification of patterns of physical activity. The ActiGraph is a small activity monitor that is used to collect and record total body physical activity, limb movements, or sleep levels. The device collects and records this information in its memory where it is then transferred from the ActiGraph onto a personal computer where the information is viewed. Its new model can collect and store activity data 24 hours a day, for up to 45 days.

Advantages and limitations: Use of a motion sensor has the advantage of relatively low cost and the generation of information on PA patterns. However, the accelerometers cannot tell the type of PA. The uniaxial accelerometer is only sensitive to movements on the vertical plan. Therefore, it is limited in its ability to detect the wide variety of movements of young children. The first generation accelerometer is also limited by possible participant tampering because of the easy accessibility to its controls, especially when applied in children. The triaxial accelerometer may have advantages over the uniaxial device, and are more likely to accurately record activities that include extensive horizontal motion. The lack of external controls also reduces the possibility of tampering. Further studies are needed on the calibration and the validation of the triaxial accelerometry and the calibration of counts against caloric cost for different free-play activities in children.

Conclusion

The development of new techniques for the assessment of PA is probably one of the most emergent needs that could benefit from incorporation of advanced technology (Goran, 1998) Clearly, there is a strong need for the development and testing of specific questionnaires for use in children, although given the constraints of this approach in general, the questionnaire approach may not be a suitable approach for assessing PA in children. The accuracy of any new questionnaire will always be limited by the ability of the subject (or the ability of his or her parents) to recall information accurately and without bias. Therefore, interview instruments should incorporate cognitive contextual cues to assist in the recollection of accurate information. In addition, because of the complex nature of PA, new techniques should provide information on the quantitative as well as the qualitative aspects (Goran, 1998). Direct observation approaches appear to offer a strong possibility for overcoming measurement issues, particularly in younger children, for whom the chances of behavioral bias might be reduced. Sophisticated techniques can be employed to address these issues. Validation of existing technology such as three dimensional accelerometry in children under a variety of conditions is also warranted. Such studies rely greatly on assessing duration, type, energy cost, efficiency, and intensity of habitual free-living activity as well as specific activities performed routinely by children. Laboratory measures of fitness and economy should be examined for their capability of predicting free-living habitual activity. Alternative noninvasive measures of muscle function and metabolism can be examined for their potential in predicting habitual PA. In addition, the assessment of PA should consider the strong likelihood of intra-individual variation (Goran, 1995) because of seasonal fluctuations, behavioral factors, and the highly volitional nature of PA. Therefore, it is important to identify the optimal period and timing of data collection.

References

Aadahl, M. & Jorgensen, T. (2003). Validation of a new self-report instrument for measuring physical activity. *Medicine & Science in Sports & Exercise*, 35: 1196–1202.

Armstrong, N. (1998). Young people's physical activity patterns as assessed by heart rate monitoring. *Journal of Sports Science*, 16: 9–16.

Berke, E.M., Gardner, A.W., Goran, M.I., & Poehlman, E.T. (1992). Resting metabolic rate and the influence of the pretesting environment. *American Journal of Clinical Nutrition*, 55: 626–629

Booth, F. W., Chakravarthy, M. V., Gordon, S. E., & Spangenburg, E. E. (2002). Waging war on physical inactivity: using modern molecular ammunition against an ancient enemy. *Journal of Applied Physiology*, 93: 3–30.

Crocker, P. R. E., Bailey, D. A., Faulkner, R. A., Kowalski, K. C., & McGrath, R. (1997). Measuring general levels of physical activity: preliminary evidence for the physical activity questionnaire for older children. *Medicine & Science in Sports & Exercise*, 29: 1344–1349.

Crouter, S. E., Schneider, P.L., Karabulut, M., & Bassett, D.R. (2003). Validity of ten electronic pedometers for measuring steps, distance, and energy cost. *Medicine & Science in Sports Exercise*, 35:1455–1460.

Cyarto, E. V., Myers, A.M., & Tudor-Locke, C. (2004). Pedometer accuracy in nursing home and community-dwelling older adults. *Medicine & Science in Sports & Exercise*, 36: 205–209.

Daniels, S. R., Morrison, J. A., Sprecher, D. L., Khoury, P., & Kimball, T. R. (1999). Association of body fat distribution and cardiovascular risk factors in children and adolescents. *Circulation*, 99: 541–545.

Figueroa-Colon, R, Franklin, F.A., Goran, M.I., Lee, J.Y., & Weinsier, R.L. (1996) Reproducibility of measurement of resting energy expenditure in prepubertal girls. *American Journal of Clinical Nutrition*, 64: 533–539.

Fu, F. H. & Hao, X. (2002). Physical development and lifestyle of Hong Kong secondary school students. *Preventive Medicine*, 35: 499–505.

Goran, M.I. (1995). Variation in total energy expenditure in humans. *Obesity Research*, 3: 59–66.

Goran, M.I. (1998). Measurement issues related to studies of childhood obesity: assessment of body composition, body fat distribution, physical activity, and food intake. *Pediatrics*, 101: 505–518.

Goran, M. I., Hunter, G., & Nagy, T. R. (1997). Physical activity related and fat mass in young children. *International Journal of Obesity*, 21, 171–178.

Goran, M. I., Poehlman, E. T., & Danforth, E. J. (1994). Experimental reliability of the doubly labeled water technique. *American Journal of Physiology*, 266, 510–515.

Gortmaker, S. L., Must, A., Sobol, A. M., Peterson, K., Colditz, G. A., & Dietz, W. H. (1996). Television viewing as a cause of increasing obesity among children in the United States, 1986–1990. *Archives of Pediatrics and Adolescent Medicine*, 150: 356–362.

Grund, A., Dilbe, B., Forberger, K., Krause, H., Siewers, M., Rieckert, H., & Muller, M. J. (2000). Relationships between physical activity, physical fitness, muscle strength and nutritional state in 5- to 11-year-old children. *European Journal of Applied Physiology*, 82: 425–438.

Horswill, C. A., Zipf, W. B., & Kien, C. L. (1997). Measuring energy costs of leisure activity in adolescents using a CO_2 breath test. *Medicine & Science in Sports Science*, 29: 1263–1268.

Janz, K. F., Levy, S. M., Burns, T. L., Torner, J. C., Willing, M. C., & Warren, J. J. (2002). Fatness, physical activity, and television viewing in children during the adiposity rebound period: the Iowa bone development study. *Preventive Medicine*, 35: 563–571.

Jones, P. J. H., Winthrop, A. L., Schoeller, D. A., Swyer, P. R., Smith, J., Filler, R. M., & Heim, T. (1987). Validation of doubly labeled water for assessing energy expenditure in infants. *Pediatric Research*, 21: 242–246.

Kilanowski, K., Angela, R. C., & Leonard, H. E. (1999). Validation of an electronic pedometer for measurement of physical activity in children, *Colleen Pediatric Exercise Science*, 11: 63–8.

Lauer, R. M. & Clarke, W. R. (1989). Childhood risk factors for high adult blood pressure: the Muscatine study. *Pediatrics*, 84: 633–641.

Le Masurier, G., Lee, S.M., & Tudor-Locke, C. (2004). Motion sensor accuracy under controlled and free-living conditions. *Medicine & Science in Sports & Exercise*, 36: 905–910.

Leung, S. S. F., Lee, W. T. K., Lui, S. S. H., Ng, M. Y., Peng, X. H., Luo, H. Y., Lam, C. W. K., & Davies, D. D. P. (2000). Fat intake in Hong Kong Chinese children. *American Journal of Clinical Nutrition*, 72: 1373–1378.

Livingstone, M.B.E., Coward, W.A., & Prentice, A.M. (1992). Daily energy expenditure in free-living children: comparison of heart- rate monitoring with the doubly labeled water $(2H^2(18)^O)$ method. *American Journal Clinical Nutrition*, 56: 343–352.

Melanson, E.L., Knoll, J.R., Bell, M.L., Donahoo, W.T., Hill, J.O., Nysse, L.J., Lanningham-Foster, L., Peters, J.C., & Levine, J.A. (2004). Commercially available pedometers: considerations for accurate step counting. *Preventive Medicine*, 39: 361–368.

Montoye, H. J., Kemper, H. C. G., Saris, W. H. M., & Washburn, R. A. (1996). *Measuring Physical Activity and Energy Expenditure*. Human Kinetics.

Murgatroyd, P. R., Shetty, P. S. & Prentice, A. M. (1993). Techniques for the measurement of human energy expenditure: a practical guide. *International Journal of Obesity*, 17: 594–568.

Patrick, L., Schneider, P.L., Crouter, S.E., & Bassett, D.R. (2004). Pedometer measures of free-living physical activity: comparison of 13 models. *Medicine & Science in Sports & Exercise*, 36: 331–335.

Robinson, T. N. (1999). Reducing children's television viewing to prevent obesity: A randomized controlled trial. *Journal of the American Medical Association*, 282: 1561–1567.

Sallis, J. F., Strikmiller, P. K., Harsha, D. W. (1996). Validation of interviewer and self-administrated physical activity checklists for fifth grade students. *Medicine & Science in Sports Exercise*, 28: 840–851.

Schneider, P.L., Crouter, S.E., Lukajic, O., & Bassett, D.R. (2003). Accuracy and reliability of 10 pedometers for measuring steps over a 400-m walk. *Medicine & Science in Sports Exercise*, 35: 1779–1784.

Schoeller, D. A., & Webb, P. (1984). Five-day comparison of the doubly labeled water method with respiratory gas exchange. *American Journal of Clinical Nutrition*, 40: 153–158.

Schoeller, D. A., & Taylor, P. B. (1987). Precision of the doubly labelled water method using the two-point calculation. *Human Nutrition: Clinical Nutrition*, 41C, 215–23.

Sirard, J. R., Melanson, E. L., & Li, L. (2000). Field evaluation of the Computer

Science and Applications, Inc. physical activity monitor. *Medicine & Science in Sports & Exercise*, 32: 695–700.

Sirard, J. R., & Pate, R. R. (2001). Physical activity assessment in children and adolescents. *Sports Medicine*, 31: 439–454.

Sung, R. Y. T., Tong, P. C. Y., Yu, C. W., Lau, P. W. C., Mok, G. T. F., Yam, M. C., Lam, P. K. W., & Chan, J. C. N. (2003). High prevalence of insulin resistance and metabolic syndrome in overweight/obese preadolescent Hong Kong Chinese children aged 9–12 years. *Diabetes Care*, 26: 250–251.

Trost, S. G., Ward, D. S., McGraw, B. & Pate, R. R. (1999). Validity of the previous day physical activity recall (PDPAR) in fifth-grade children. *Pediatric Exercise Science*, 11: 341–348.

World Health Organisation. (2002). *The World Health Report: Reducing Risks, Promoting Health Life.*

Wuest, D. A. & Bucher, C. A. (2003). Foundations of Physical Education, Exercise Science, and Sport (14th ed.). *Dubuque, IA: WCB/McGraw Hill.*

Yu, C.W., Sung, R.Y.T., So, R., Lam, K., Nelson, E.A.S., Li, A.M.C., Yuan, Y., & Lam, P.K.W. (2002). Energy expenditure and physical activity of obese children: cross-sectional study. *Hong Kong Medical Journal*, 8: 313–317.

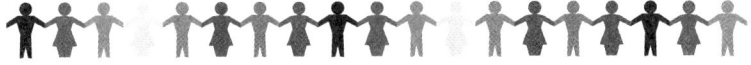

CHAPTER 3

Measuring Health-related Physical Fitness in Hong Kong Children and Youth

Stanley Sai-chuen Hui

Introduction

Periodic evaluation of health-related physical fitness in children has gained popularity in schools in most nations since the 1970s. It is believed that the profiles and changes of health-related physical fitness in children reflect the effectiveness of the physical education and sports curricula, as well as the lifestyle of children and efforts of health promotion provided by the society. Health-related physical fitness is the optimal physical capability to carry out daily activities efficiently and to allow one to resist sickness. Such physical qualities include cardio-respiratory fitness, muscular strength and endurance, musculo-skeletal flexibility, and body composition. Health-related physical fitness assessment itself can also be a useful motivational strategy to encourage regular participation in exercise training (Franks, 1997). Over the past few decades several health-related fitness batteries have been developed in western countries adopting slightly different test items. Several Asia-Pacific countries have also implemented health-related physical fitness batteries in recent years, in the form of fitness award schemes or annual fitness assessment as part of the school P.E. curriculum. With the increasing popularity of health-related physical fitness, the test items have experienced significant changes and improvement in terms of test administration, protocol selection, and validity. In this chapter a brief review is presented on the development of health-related physical fitness. Issues pertaining to the rationales and objectives of conducting health-related physical fitness evaluation will be addressed. Various protocols and test batteries will be compared. Recent development and concerns in test item selection will also be illustrated. The chapter will end by describing the health-related physical fitness profiles of Hong Kong children and youth derived from a recent cross-sectional fitness survey.

Development of Health-related Physical Fitness Evaluation for Children

Only limited literature is available documenting the development of physical fitness assessment. Perhaps body composition measurement is one of the oldest forms of assessment, known as anthropometry found in ancient cultures of Egypt, India, and Greece (Tritschler, 2000). Ancient Egyptians suggested that the "ideal" body structure is characterized by having a knee height that should be five-finger lengths (middle-finger) from the ground, whereas "one's arm-reach should be eight finger lengths". Interestingly, from empirical observation, most of the Chinese people are much shorter than the "ideal" stature suggested by ancient Egyptians. In China, the earliest form of physical fitness evaluation dates back to the Zhou Dynasty (11th–7th centuries B.C.) when Chinese people were being selected for military service. However, not until the Tang Dynasty (A.D. 702) has physical fitness screening been formalized as an imperial cadet examination, establishing a precedent of selecting elite performers. Most fitness tests were military-specific skills and abilities such as archery, chariot racing, strength tests, and martial arts. Such practice had been implemented throughout the Chinese history until the last century in the Qing Dynasty (A.D. 1644–1911). Formal physical fitness training and assessment were not common at the community level. Until the 1890s, under the influence of Western religious bodies which set up a number of Christian missionary schools, such as the Young Men's Christian Association (YMCA) and the Young Women's Christian Association (YWCA), systematic training on physical fitness and physical education using Western theory had not been imposed at the school level (Knuttgen, Ma, & Wu, 1990). Some forms of physical fitness assessments were introduced to schools but did not gain popularity. The objective of fitness assessment was selecting elite athletes for sports competition, rather than health and fitness promotion as recommended nowadays. Perhaps the first systematic large-scale physical fitness assessment was a fitness evaluation program initiated by Kraus and Hirschland (1954) after the World War II. In this project physical fitness profiles of American children were compared to those of European children. One major finding in this project was that the fitness profiles of American children were far poorer than their European counterparts. However, in this large-scale fitness project, the Kraus-Weber Test was adopted which was originally designed for measuring muscular fitness. The impact of the result was strong enough to induce US President Eisenhower to strongly support children's fitness evaluation programmes. Subsequently the American Association (now Alliance) for Health, Physical Education, and Recreation (AAHPER) *Youth Fitness Test* was established in 1958. In the 1970s, the American Alliance for Health, Physical Education, Recreation and Dance (AAHPERD) began to promote a more comprehensive concept of physical fitness, which stressed the importance of health-related components. The AAHPERD Health-related Physical Fitness Test was developed comprising components measuring cardio-respiratory function, body composition, and musculo-skeletal function (AAHPERD, 1980). Test items included one-mile run, triceps and calf skinfold thickness, sit-and-reach test, and sit-up test. In Hong Kong, few studies have reported health-related physical fitness profiles of Hong Kong school children and youth. Only three large-scale fitness assessment projects were found for school children and youth in Hong Kong. These studies were conducted by To (1985), Fu (1994), and Hui, Chan, Wong, et al. (2001a).

In 1981–1982, a cooperative cross-disciplinary research project on physical activities and quality of life was initiated by the Chinese University of Hong Kong and the University of Michigan (To et al., 1985). The Asian Committee for Standardization of Physical Fitness Test (ACSPFT) battery was administered to a representative sample of 9770 male and female Hong Kong school children, ages 9 to 18. A total of 10 physical fitness measures were obtained (Table 1). Power

Table 1. Physical fitness test items adopted by three major school fitness surveys in Hong Kong from 1985 to 2001

	To et al. (1985)	Fu et al. (1994)	Hui et al. (2001)
Power	• 50m dash • Shuttle-run • Standing long jump	—	—
Aerobic Endurance	• 1000m run for boys, 800m for girls, and 600m for under 11 years-old	• 800m run for the primary and 1600m run for the secondary school students	• 1600m run for primary 4 to form 7 students
Body Composition	• Height & weight	• Height & weight • Triceps & calf skinfolds	• Height & weight • Triceps & calf skinfolds
Muscular Strength & Endurance	• Pull-up for boys • Flexed-arm hang for girls and boys under 11 • Sit-up • Handgrip	• Sit-ups • Inclined pull-up	• Push-up for boys and modified push-up for girls • Cadence curl-up
Flexibility	• Trunk-forward flexion	• Sit and reach	• CUHK sit-and-reach

(Adapted from Hui, S.C. (2005). Manual of Health-related Physical Fitness Assessment for Hong Kong Students, Department of Sports Science and Physical Education, The Chinese University of Hong Kong)

was included as a major component in To's (1985) study which made it more a test of performance-related fitness than one of health-related fitness. Another investigation was conducted by Fu in 1990–1991 (Fu, 1994). Instead of the ACSPFT battery, this investigation adopted the International Council for Health, Physical Education and Recreation (ICHPER) *Asian Health-related Youth Fitness Test* (Hatano, 1994). This test measures 6 items (triceps skinfold, calf skinfold, 60 seconds sit-up, inclined pull-up, sit and reach, and 0.5-mile run for the primary and 1-mile run for the secondary school students). The 60-second flexed knee sit-ups test adopted in both the To and Fu studies were questioned by several critics of its validity and safety limitations (Diener 1995; Jette, Sidney, & Cicutti, 1984; Liemohn, Snodgrass, & Sharpe, 1988; Plowman 1992; Safrit, Zhu, & Costa, 1992). The traditional sit-and-reach test adopted in Fu's study was also questioned by Cailliet (1998) on the safety issue of placing too much stress on the vertebrae. Pursuant to recent investigations on improving the safety and validity of the test items, the Chinese University of Hong Kong proposed a new health-related test battery in 2001. These test items include the 1-mile run, push-up test, cadence curl-up test, triceps and calf skinfolds, and the CUHK sit-and-reach test (i.e. the modified back-saver sit-and-reach test). Over 10,000 primary and secondary school children in Hong Kong were tested from 2001 to 2002 and normative data were generated from this study (Tables 5–15 in Appendix 2 to this chapter).

Through the effort of these large-scale fitness evaluation projects, health-related fitness assessment has gained recognition in recent years from school teachers and policy makers in Hong Kong with regards to its importance to personal health, physical growth and development of school children. Several fitness assessment projects in the form of award schemes are being implemented, such as the Childhealth Foundation Fitness Award Scheme, and the Po Leung Kuk Fitness Award Scheme. Although health-related fitness assessment has gradually gained in popularity in schools of Hong Kong, further effort is still needed to develop more practical tests with improved validity and reliability. Cross-sectional data are available, but longitudinal data on changes in health-related fitness profiles are still needed. Standardization of fitness test items is also an important area of study so that cross-cultural comparisons can be made. Another important trend to note is that, while Hong Kong is catching up with the promotion of health-related fitness, current focus has been put on the promotion of regular physical activity. As a result from the 1996 *US Surgeon Generals' Report on Physical Activity and Health* (U.S. Department of Health and Human Services,USDHHS, 1996), the goal of exercise promotion has been switched from fitness to activity. Exercise prescription used to focus on quality (a certain level of exercise intensity) but now more on the quantity (total daily energy expenditure or exercise duration). In the year 2000, a more specific report related to physical activity promotion for children and youth was released by the USDHHS. The FITNESSGRAM, one of the most widely promoted fitness scheme in the US for over 20 years, has stressed the importance of physical activity measurement and incorporated physical activity as one of the elements being evaluated (Cooper Institute for Aerobics Research, CIAR, 1999).

Rationale and Objectives

Components of health-related fitness tests include cardio-respiratory function in terms of aerobic capacity, body composition particularly the ratio of body fatness to body mass, and musculo-skeletal function including strength, endurance, and flexibility. Rationale for the inclusion of these items is based on the belief that these fitness components are highly related to personal health status. Through assessment of health-related fitness, individuals with a poor fitness level can be identified so that appropriate exercise prescription can be provided to improve their fitness and health conditions. Some individuals can be motivated to exercise simply by taking the fitness assessments. Coaches and teachers often administered fitness tests before and after a physical conditioning period so as to evaluate the effectiveness of the program from the changes in fitness levels. Some teachers adopt fitness tests as criterion measures for grade determination. This brings up the controversial question whether personal fitness level should be used for grading purposes. The argument is that some scientists believe that fitness should be promoted and compared on a personal basis and should not be compared inter-personally. For example, a student should not get a higher grade because his/her body fat is less than other students. Although body fatness is partly attributed to sedentary lifestyle and unhealthy diet, other strong confounding factors such as heredity and parental influence are out of the student's control. Moreover, since the criteria for grading are usually based on normative data collected from the same population, the rationale for giving students a specific grade (such as C) for a certain percentile rank (such as 50 percentile) is not justifiable. Recently, scientists have suggested that the criteria for fitness evaluation should be based upon a minimum health-related standard, and only a pass/fail grade should be given to students who meet/do not meet the minimum health standard. For example, Blair, Kohl, Paffenbarger, et al. (1989) suggested that the minimum health standard for aerobic fitness is 35 ml/kg/min for men and 32.5 ml/kg/min for women. FITNESSGRAM (CIAR, 1999) recommends a score of 8 inches on the Back-saver Sit-and-reach test be considered a 'pass' for all boys. Nevertheless, if performance in fitness assessment is used for grading purposes, then reasonable objectives should be clearly identified at the beginning of the training period and appropriate amount of time should be provided for achieving the objectives.

Aerobic capacity is one of the most important elements in health-related fitness. Other terms such as cadiorespiratory endurance, cardiovascular fitness, and aerobic power have been used as synonyms. It is well documented that levels of aerobic capacity are associated with a reduced risk of coronary heart disease, high blood pressure, obesity, diabetes, and some kind of cancer (Blair et al. 1989; Blair, Kohl, Gordon, et al., 1992; USDHHS, 1996). Ideally, the level of aerobic capacity is evaluated in terms of a maximal oxygen consumption (VO2max). However, the direct measure of maximal oxygen consumption requires participants to exercise to exhaustion. The associated risk and the required sophisticated metabolic measuring equipment make this test not feasible for mass and field testing, especially for testing children. Field tests, such as running and walking tests, have been reported to be highly correlated to VO2max. Therefore, these field tests are widely adopted in schools for evaluating aerobic capacity. However, the measuring outcome is usually the performance time covering a certain distance, or the distance being covered within a certain time period, instead of the gold standard VO2max.

Muscular strength, muscular endurance, and flexibility are important aspects that influence muscular-skeletal function. Poor muscular strength and endurance are associated with increased risk of injuries and inability of performing daily lifting tasks. These muscular fitness components are also essential for high-level performance in many sports. Good muscular strength is also important for maintaining good posture, which would help to prevent sagging abdominal muscles and low-back pain. Good muscular endurance enables individuals to perform repeated muscular activities more efficiently, such as walking stairs and arm strokes in swimming. Low back pain, which is increasingly common in modern society, is associated with poor abdominal muscle tone and poor flexibility of the lower back and hamstring muscles. Poor flexibility in the back can be responsible for poor posture, compression of nerves around lumbar region, painful menstruation, and other body ailments. Poor flexibility is also characterized by a lack of muscular elasticity and a limitation of joint mobility, which would result from injury during rapid or forceful muscular exertion.

Body composition, particularly the relative fat contents in the body compared to body mass, perhaps is the next most important aspects in health-related fitness after aerobic capacity. Excessive body fat has been associated with a number of health problems such as diabetes, coronary heart disease, stroke, and hypertension. The measurement of body composition has increasingly been viewed as important in children nowadays. The 2000 USDHHS report revealed that obesity in children and youth has risen to an alarming extent. Overweight in adolescence increased from 5.4% to 9.7% in girls and 4.5% to 11.3% in boys, from the years 1976–80 to 1988–94. In Hong Kong, as in other urbanized cities, the overweight problem in children is on the rise. In 1993, 10–13% of children and youth in Hong Kong aged 6 to18 years were classified as being obese (Leung, Ng, & Lau, 1995). By 1998, 23% of boys and 10% of girls age 9 to 12 years were obese (Guldan, Cheung, & Chui, 1998). Overweight children are deemed to have poor self-esteem and become obese in adulthood. Periodic evaluation of body fatness is important so that overly fat children can be identified and receive timely and appropriate treatment such as a combination of exercise and diet control.

Selection of Fitness Test Items

To effectively evaluate fitness of children, the selection of appropriate test items is a concern. Principles of reliability, validity, practicality should be emphasized when selecting testing items. Table 2 summarizes

Table 2. Comparison of Various Health-related Fitness Test Protocols

Fitness Components	FITNESS-GRAM	President's Challenge	NCYFS	Taiwan	China	HK Child health/ED	PLK	AYP	HKCEE	CUHK
CV Fitness	1-mile for 10–18, no time standard for 5–9	1-mile run for 10 above, 0.25 mile for 6–7, 0.5 mile for 8–9	1-mile run for 8 above, 0.5 mile for 6–7	1600m for secondary boys, 800m for all girls and p.3–p.6 boys	9' & 12' run	6' & 9' run/walk	1000m (boys), 800m (girls)	800m	1-mile run	1-mile run
Muscular Endurance	Curl-up	Curl-up	1-min sit-up	1-min sit-up	1-min sit-up	1-min sit-up	30s sit-up, 30s Bailey Bridge	1-min sit-up, 30s Bailey Bridge	1-min sit-up	GT curl-up
Muscular Strength	Push-up	Pull-up, push-up	Pull-up	—	Handgrip, flex-arm hang, pull-up	Handgrip, push-up	Handgrip	Push-up	Pull-up (boys), flex-arm hang (girls)	Push-up
Flexibility	Back-saver	Sit-reach	Sit-reach	Sit-reach	Sit-reach	Sit-reach	Sit-reach		Sit-reach	CUHK Sit-reach
Body Composition	Triceps+ Calf	BMI	Triceps+ Calf	BMI	Triceps+ Subscapular skinfolds	Triceps+ Calf skinfolds	—	—	—	Triceps+ Calf

Remarks:

AYP – Award for Young People Fitness Testing Scheme

China – China National Children and Youth Fitness Assessment System (National Sports Council of China, 2000)

CUHK – Cross-sectional Fitness Survey conducted by the Department of Sports Science and P.E., The Chinese U. of Hong Kong

FITNESSGRAM – A nationwide fitness award scheme for primary and secondary schools in the US.

HKCEE – Hong Kong Certificate of Education Examination, Fitness Components of P.E. examination

HK Childhealth/ED – Hong Kong Childhealth Foundation/Education Department Physical Fitness Award Scheme

NCYFS – National Children and Youth Fitness Survey, US, 1985

President's Challenge – President's Challenge Physical Fitness Award Scheme, a nationwide fitness award scheme for the publics, US

PLK – Po Leung Kuk Schools Physical Fitness Award Scheme

Taiwan – Taiwan Annual Physical Fitness Evaluation Scheme, National Council of Physical Fitness and Sports testing items adopted in several large-scale fitness testing protocols in Hong Kong, compared with nation-wide fitness assessment protocols in the USA and Taiwan. As can be seen, considerable discrepancy in test selection exists among these protocols. There are a number of pros and cons for each protocol. In general, most fitness items demonstrate good to high reliability. Some tests possess satisfactory validity but in others validity is just fair. For aerobic capacity, all protocols have adopted running tests but vary in required distance or time. However, the criterion-related validity of most running test has not been documented for children and youth. The rationale for adopting a running test is its logical validity. The 1-mile run test has been adopted in most nationwide fitness test batteries including those of the USA and Taiwan, except for girls inTaiwan who run the 800M test. The advantage of using a 1-mile run is that normative data and health-related standards have been published so that comparisons can easily be made.

Educators may utilize these comparisons to evaluate the physical growth and changes in fitness levels of children. One drawback of the 1-mile run is that it may be too long a distance for primary school students aged 9 years or younger. However, no matter what distance is selected, the difficulty in motivating such young children to perform a maximal run hinders the value of assessing true aerobic fitness in this manner. Therefore, as recommended by FITNESSGRAM and the President's Council for Physical Fitness, young children of 9 years-old or under should be encouraged to participate in run test but no time standard should be determined for them. The problem with the 800M run is that it has been viewed as a middle-distance running test that requires a combination of aerobic and anaerobic power, and therefore not truly representing the cardio-respiratory endurance.

As for muscular fitness, Table 2 indicates that most fitness batteries in Hong Kong have adopted the traditional 1-min flexed leg sit-up speed test to evaluate "abdominal muscle strength and endurance". This 1-min sit-up test is similar to the AAHPERD (1980) sit-up test. In essence, a one-minute, bent-knee sit-up test with feet anchored, is a test for muscular power instead of strength and endurance. Recent studies suggest uncertainty about its safety and validity, and this kind of sit-up test is no longer the choice for evaluating abdominal fitness

(Jette et al., 1984; Liemohn et al., 1988; Plowman, 1992). Cadence testing, such as the Georgia-Tech University Curl-up Test, which uses a standard cadence (e.g. 25/min.) for cueing sit-ups, greatly reduces undue stress in the lower back, bouncing and jarring movements and possible abdominal injuries as in the "speed test" in the past years (Quinney, Smith, & Wenger, 1984; Sparling, 1997). Furthermore, the cadence test was proven to measure one dimension of abdominal muscular endurance, while speed tests measure a different dimension of abdominal fitness (CIAR, 1999 ; Diener, 1995; Jette et al., 1984, Safrit, 1992).

In many of the older tests, the pull-up was usually used for boys and flexed-arm-hang for girls for testing upper body strength. Both of these tests have significant drawbacks. In many cases, subjects are not able to sustain even one pull-up or a single second of flexed arm hanging, thus rendering the measurement invalid. Even for subjects who are able to do more than one pull-up, the limited number of successful pull-ups reduces the predictability of strength level of participants. Recently, scientists suggest that the push-up test for boys and the modified push-up (on knees) for girls are still the most practical field tests for measuring upper limb strength and endurance. The push-up ensures at least a moderate success rate for most participants and thus enhances the value in making comparisons. The Prudential FITNESSGRAM and the CUHK fitness test battery have adopted the push-up test.

With regard to flexibility, the modified back-saver Sit-and-Reach Test (i.e., the CUHK Sit-and-Reach test) has been considered the safest sit-and-reach test, with better validity and reliability (CIAR, 1999, Heyward, 2002; Hui & Yuen, 2000) among existing protocols. The traditional sit-and-reach test requires participants to straighten both legs with feet against a sit-and-reach box while sitting on the floor. This test has been criticised in that it places undesirable strain on the lower vertebrae when reaching forward and results in excessive posterior disc compression due to the anterior portion of the vertebrae being pressed together (Cailliet, 1988). In other words, repeated performance of the traditional sit-and-reach test may have detrimental effects on lower back health. The CUHK Sit-and-Reach Test has been recommended because of its protective effects on lower back vertebrae and muscles. Moreover, it does not require a sit-and-reach box as in the original modified back-saver sit-and-reach test. Only a 12-inches high bench and a 1-meter measuring tape are needed. Research indicated that participants preferred CUHK sit-and-reach test over other similar protocols because it is a more comfortable test (Hui & Yuen, 2000).

For body composition, skinfold measurements comprise an excellent field test for assessing subcutaneous fat. Evaluation of body composition using height-weight table or body mass index (BMI) is not ideal, as no estimation of percent body fat can be made. Janz, Nielsen, Cazssidy, et al. (1993) studied various skinfold measurement methods for children and youth, and concluded that the triceps and subscapular measures are the most accurate among those methods that use only two sites. Yet, Heyward and Stolarczyk (1998) suggested that in consideration of the sensitivity and ethical issues regarding physical contact with children, triceps and calf measuring sites (Slaughter, Lohman, Boileau, et al., 1988) are a more suitable choice, although accuracy is slightly affected. Most modern mass testing protocols for youth adopt this method. However, cross-validation of the 2-site formula on Chinese children and youth in Hong Kong has not been well established. Hui, Chan, Wong, et al. (2001b) cross-validated the Slaughter 2-site formula on 141 Hong Kong children age 8 to 13 year-old and found that the equation consistently over-estimated body fat with larger errors. Hui et al. (2001b) suggested that only the triceps skinfold for boys (%fat=−0.31+1.481*triceps; R^2=.68, SEE=5.18%) and only the calf skinfold for girls (%fat=2.577+ 1.277*calf; R^2=.53, SEE=5.07%) would yield satisfactory estimation of percent body fat for Chinese children. Further effort is needed to develop validated skinfold equations for estimating percent fat that cover a wider age range of Hong Kong children (e.g. from 8 to 18 years).

Profiles of Health-related Fitness of Hong Kong Children and Youth

With the support from the University Grants Council of Hong Kong, the Chinese University of Hong Kong (CUHK) has conducted a large-scale health-related physical fitness and activity survey in year 2000–2001. Over 10,000 students from primary 4 to form 7 from 37 schools

(17 primary, 20 secondary) were tested and the testing items selected were slightly different from previous studies in Hong Kong (To et al., 1985; Fu, 1994). A summary of the test descriptions of the CUHK health-related fitness test battery is presented on Table 4 (Appendix 1 to this chapter). The tests items were published in various reports which indicated excellent validity, these items included 1-mile run/walk for aerobic fitness (AAHPERD, 1984; Cureton & Warren, 1990), CUHK sit-and-reach test for flexibility (Hui & Yuen, 2000), push-up test for upper body strength and endurance (American College of Sports Medicine [ACSM], 2000), GT cadence curl-up test for trunk strength and endurance (Sparling, 1997), and 2-site (triceps and calf) skinfolds for body fat estimation (Slaughter et al., 1988). The test battery was similar to that adopted by the FITNESSGRAM except that the latter adopted the feet-on-floor (bent-knee) cadence curl-up and the original back-saver sit-and-reach test. Boys accounted for 46.7% of the sample, girls for 53.3%. The distributions in gender, grade levels, school districts, and school types were very similar to the 1999 report of the Education Department.

Normative results, in terms of percentile ranks and quintile categories, by age and gender are displayed in Table 5 to 16 (Appendix 2 to this chapter). Overall speaking, health-related fitness of boys was significantly better than girls. The mean 1-mile run time for boys was 9.4 minutes, which was 1.7 minute faster than girls (11.1 min). The mean curl-up for boys was 23.1 reps, which was approximately 4 reps more than girls (18.9 reps). The sum of triceps and calf skinfolds of boys (24.2 mm) were 6.5 mm less than girls (30.7 mm). However, the low-back and hamstrings flexibilities of girls were much better than boys (right leg:57.3 cm vs 53.2 cm; left leg: 56.7 cm vs 52.5 cm). The trends of better aerobic fitness, muscular endurance, and body composition, and poorer flexibilities in boys, as compared to girls, were consistent across different age groups. The patterns of changes in different fitness components were different. Results also indicated that most health-related fitness improved in S-shape as age increase. Most fitness parameters improved with age in S-shape, except the curl-up performance of boys was in inverted-U shape where the best performance occurred at age 15.

When the physical fitness performance of this Hong Kong sample

Table 3. Comparison of passing rates of Hong Kong students to US
          students

	1-mile Run	Push-up	Curl-up	SR-right	SR-left	Skinfolds
HK-girls	49.7%	87.6%	56.7%	65.4%	63%	88%
US- girls[1]	60%	32%	N.A. [2]	97%	97%	91%
HK-boys	65.4%	62.2%	55.6%	72.9%	70%	79.7%
US-boys[1]	77%	73%	N.A. [2]	90%	90%	89%

Notes:
1. Data from Looney & Plowman (1990).
2. Curl-up passing rates of American children were not available.

was compared to the health standards published by the FITNESSGRAM (CIAR, 1999), only half (49.7%) of girls and 65.4% of boys met the aerobic fitness criteria. For muscular fitness of the girls, 87.6% passed the push-up and only 56.7% passed the curl-up tests. For the boys, only 62.2% passed the push-up and 55.6% passed the curl-up test. For flexibility, slightly more than 60% of the girls and more than 70% of the boys passed the sit-and-reach tests. For body composition, 79.7% of the boys and 88% of the girls passed the skinfold thickness standards. When these passing rates were compared to those obtained for US students from the data of 1985 and 1987 national surveys (Looney & Plowman, 1990), as summarized in Table 3, Hong Kong students demonstrated lower passing rates in general. These results suggested that the health-related physical fitness profiles of Hong Kong students were poorer than US students. Based upon the results of this study, it is suggested that physical fitness enhancement programs for Hong Kong students be strengthened.

Conclusion

Health-related fitness promotion for children and youth is gaining in popularity due to its strong association with health improvement and maintenance. Periodic assessment of health-related fitness provides quantitative information for teachers, coaches and parents to understand the physical growth, changes and profiles of children. Such information may also reflect the effectiveness of the physical education curriculum in schools, as well as exercise promotion provided by the community. Health-related fitness profiles also reflect the effectiveness of society as a whole in how well it cultivates children who reside in the community. Hong Kong is a highly urbanized and modernized city. The advances in facilities and living environment reduce the need and opportunities for children to be active at home, school or even at the outdoor environment. Food is abundant in most families. The number of fast-food restaurants increase rapidly and they are gaining popularity with the children. The increase in childhood obesity in Hong Kong is now a concern. To combat the impact of an inactive lifestyle and unhealthy diet, the physical education curriculum plays an important role in educating the correct concepts of staying fit and healthy through active participation in sport and exercise. To evaluate how well the physical education curriculum promotes fitness and health, assessment of health-related fitness of children becomes important, even necessary. In Hong Kong, several fitness testing schemes have been lauched in the past decade, but different testing items were adopted. Moreover, most of these studies were cross-sectional. Longitudinal changes in fitness conditions are still not documented. Although some studies involved slightly more than ten thousand subjects, citywide fitness evaluation on a much larger scale is needed in order to better understand the fitness profiles of children and youth. Such evaluation is to be carried out annually and changes in physical fitness conditions have to be examined. To achieve such a purpose, the standardization of fitness testing items becomes a necessity for frequent testing to be administered among different schools and districts, and would provide for cross-cultural comparisons. Efforts are still needed to develop more practical tests with improved reliability and validity of testing protocols.

References

American Alliance for Health, Physical Education, Recreation and Dance (AAHPERD). (1980). *AAHPERD Health-related Physical Fitness Test manual.* Reston, VA: Author.

AAHPERD (1984). Technical manual: Health-related physical fitness. Reston, VA: Author.

American College of Sports Medicine (2000). *Guidelines for exercise testing and prescription (6th ed.)*. Media, PA: Lippincott Williams & Wilkins.

Blair, S. N., Kohl, H. W., Gordon, N.F., & Paffenbarger, R. S., Jr., (1992). How much physical activity is good for health? *Annals and Reviews in Public Health, 13,* 99–126.

Blair, S. N., Kohl, H. W., Paffenbarger, R. S., Jr., Clark, D. G., Cooper, K. H., & Gibbons, L. W. (1989). Physical fitness and all-cause mortality: A prospective study of healthy men and women. *Journal of the American Medical Association, 262,* 2395–2437.

Cailliet, R. (1988). *Low back pain syndrome (4th ed.)*. Philadelphia: F.A. Davis Company.

Cooper Institute for Aerobics Research (1999). *The Prudential FITNESSGRAM Test administration manual*. Dallas, Texas: Author.

Cureton, K. J., Warren, G. L. (1990). Criterion-referenced standards for youth health-related fitness tests: A tutorial. *Research Quarterly for Exercise and Sport, 61,* 7–19.

Diener, M. H., Golding, L. A., & Diener, D. (1995). Validity and reliability of a one-minute half sit-up test of abdominal strength and endurance. *Sports Medicine, Training and Rehabilitation, 6,* 105–119.

Education Department (1999). *Enrolment statistics 1998*. Hong Kong: Education Department Statistics Section.

Franks, B. D. (1997). Move it kids: Evaluating physical activity and fitness in children and youth. *American College of Sports Medicine's Health & Fitness Journal, 1,* 20–24.

Fu, F. H. (1994). *Health fitness parameters of Hong Kong school children*. Hong Kong: Department of Physical Education, Hong Kong Baptist College.

Guldan, G. S., Cheung, I. L. T., Chui, K. K. H. (1998). Childhood obesity in Hong Kong: embracing an unhealthy lifestyle before puberty. *International Journal of Obesity, 22*(Suppl. 4): S49.

Hatano, Y. (1994). ICHPERD.SD Asia Youth Health Related Fitness Test: Construction of norms for Japanese students. *ICHPERD.SD Journal, 30,* 8–15.

Heyward. V. H. (2002). *Advanced fitness assessment and exercise prescription (4th. ed.)*. Champaign, IL: Human Kinetics.

Heyward, V. H., & Stolarczyk, L. M. (1996). *Applied body composition assessment*. Champaign, IL: Human Kinetics.

Hui, S.C. (2005). *Manual of Health-related Physical Fitness Assessment for Hong*

Kong Students. Department of Sports Science and Physical Education, The Chinese University of Hong Kong

Hui, S. C., Chan, C. M., Wong, S. H. S., Ha, A. S. C., & Hong, Y. (2001). Physical activity level of Chinese youths and its association with physical fitness and demographic variables: The Hong Kong Youth Fitness Study. *Research Quarterly for Exercise and Sport, 72*(supplement), A92–93.

Hui, S. C., Chan, W. S., Wong, H. S. S., Wong, G. W. K., & Lau, W. C. (2001). Evaluation of skinfolds measurement in estimating body fat of Chinese children. *Medicine and Science in Sports and Exercise, 33*(5) (supplement), S244, #1369.

Hui, S. C., & Yuen, P. Y. (2000). Validity of the Modified Back Saver Sit-And-Reach Test: A comparison with other protocols. *Medicine and Science in Sports and Exercise, 32*, 1655–1659.

Janz, K. F., Nielsen, D. H., Cassady, S. L., Cook, J. S., Wu, Y., & Hansen, J. R. (1993). Cross-validation of the Slaughter skinfold equations for children and adolescents. *Medicine and Science in Sports and Exercise, 25*, 1070–1076.

Jette, M., K. Sidney, M., & Cicutti, . (1984). A critical analysis of sit-ups: A case for the partial curl as a test of abdominal muscular endurance. *Canadian Alliance of Health, Physical Education and Recreation Journal, 51*, 4–9.

Knuttgen, H. G., Ma, Q. W., & Wu, Z. Y. (1990). *Sport in China.* Champaign, IL: Human Kinetics.

Kraus, H., & Hirschland, R. P. (1954). Minimum muscular fitness test in school children. *Research Quarterly, 25*, 177–188.

Leung, S. S. F., Ng, M. Y., Lau, T. F. (1995). Prevalence of obesity in Hong Kong children and adolescents aged 3-18 years. *Chinese Journal of Preventive Medicine, 29*, 270–272.

Liemohn, W., Snodgrass, L. B., & Sharpe, G. L. (1988). Unresolved controversies in back management: A review. *Journal of Orthopedic and Sports Physical Therapy, 9*, 239–244.

Looney, M. A., & Plowman, S. A. (1990). Passing rates of American children and youth on the FITNESSGRAM criterion-referenced physical fitness standards. *Research Quarterly for Exercise and Sport, 61*, 215–223

National Sports Council of China (2000). Study of physical fitness of citizens in China. Beijing, China: Beijing University of Physical Education Press.

Plowman, S. A. (1992). Physical activity, physical fitness, and low back pain. In J. O. Holloszy (Ed.), *Exercise and sport science reviews* (pp. 221–224). Baltimore MD: Williams & Wilkens.

Safrit, M. J., Zhu, W., & Costa, M. G. (1992). The difficulty of sit-up tests: An empirical investigation. *Research Quarterly for Exercise and Sport, 68,* 80–84.

Slaughter, M. H., Lohman, T. G., Boileau, R. A., Horswill, C. A., Stillman, R. J., Van Loan, M. D., & Bemben, D. A. (1988). Skinfold equations for estimation of body fatness in children and youth. *Human Biology, 60,* 709–723.

Sparling, P. B. (1997). Field testing for abdominal muscular fitness: Speed versus cadence sit-ups. *ACSM'S Health & Fitness Journal, 1,* 30–33.

To, C. Y. (1985). *Physical fitness of children in Hong Kong.* Hong Kong: The Chinese University of Hong Kong, School of Education.

Tritschler, K. (2000). Barrow & McGee's Practical Measurement and Assessment (5th Ed.). Philadelphia, PA: Lippincott Williams & Wilkins, pp. 27.

U.S. Department of Health and Human Services. (1996). *Physical activity and health: A report of the Surgeon General.* Atlanta, GA: U.S. Department of Health and Human Services, Centers for Disease Control and Prevention, National Center for Chronic Disease Prevention and Health Promotion.

U. S. Department of Health and Human Services. (2000). *Promoting better health for young people through physical activity and sports: A report to the President from the Secretary of Health and Human Services and the Secretary of Education.* Atlanta, GA: U.S. Department of Health and Human Services, Centers for Disease Control and Prevention, National Center for Chronic Disease Prevention and Health Promotion.

Appendix 1. The CUHK Health-related Fitness Test

Table 4. *The CUHK Health-related Fitness Test*
(Reprinted from Hui et al., 2005)

Test	Description	
One-mile Run	Objective	Assessing aerobic capacity
	Equipment	Stop watch and a 1-mile (1609m) distance jogging track (such as a 400-meter track or a basketball court, to count the number of laps that children run to accumulate the 1-mile distance)
	Instructions	Assign students to work in pairs. One as runner and the other as time keeper. Runner gets ready in front of the starting line and time keeper holds a stop watch for keeping the time. At the signals of "Ready! Go!", time keeper starts the stop watch and runner runs, or jogs, or walks as fast as possible to cover the 1-mile distance. To ensure a valid test, runner should try his/her best effort to cover the 1-mile distance with the shortest time. Although runner is allowed to jog and even walk whenever they feel tired during the test, they should run again whenever they feel capable. When runner passes the finishing line, time keeper stops the stop watch. The time in minutes and seconds is the score of the runner. After sufficient rest, runner and time keeper switch positions.
Cadence Curl-up	Objective	Assessing muscular strength and endurance
	Equipment	Metronome (optional but recommended), safety mat, bench (approximately 12" high)
	Instructions	Assign students to work in pairs. One as testee and the other as tester. Testee lies on floor in a supine position. Feet placed on a 12" high bench with thigh perpendicular to the floor. Arms cross on chest. A metronome is used for controlling the rhythm of curl-up movement at a speed of 25 curl-up per minute. If metronome

		is not available, instruct testee to perform one curl-up every 2–3 second. At the signal of "Ready? Go!", testee performs as many curl-up as possible at a steady speed. A successful repetition is counted when elbow touches the mid-thigh and then the upper back touches the floor. There is no time limit but testee has to perform curl-up continuously at a constant rhythm. If the testee fails to perform a standard movement but the movement is performed continuously, then the testee is allowed to continue with the test but that repetition is not counted. Tester counts the number of successful repetitions as the performance score of the testee.
		Preparation position Standard posture of a successful curl-up
Push-up	Objective	Assessing muscular strength and endurance of boys
	Equipment	Safety mat
	Instructions	Assign students to work in pairs. One as testee and the other as tester. Testee prepares at a prone position on the safety mat as shown below. Body supports by both hands and feet. At the signal of "Ready! Go!", testee performs as many push-up as possible at a steady speed (about 2–3 seconds per repetition). There is no time limit but testee has to perform push-up continuously. Once there is pause in movement, the test stopped. A successful repetition is counted when elbow is flexed at $90°$ and then straightens again. If the testee fails to perform a standard form of movement but the

		movement is performed continuously, then the testee is allowed to continue with the test but that repetition is not counted. Tester counts the number of successful repetitions as the performance score of the testee.
		Preparation position Standard posture of a successful push-up
Modified Push-up	Objective	For assessing muscular strength and endurance of girls
	Equipment	Safety mat
	Instructions	Same as push-up test for boy, except that girl is prone on safety mat with both hands and knees supporting the body. Preparation position Standard posture of a successful push-up
CUHK Sit-and-Reach	Objective	Assessing flexibility
	Equipment	Bench (approximately 12" high), a 1-meter measuring tape
	Instructions	Assign students to work in pairs. One as testee and the other as tester. Unlike traditional sit-and-reach test, sit-and-reach box is not required in this test. Testee sits on the bench with one leg straight on bench. A 1-meter measuring tape is placed on the bench with the marking of 50 cm

<table>
<tr><td></td><td></td><td>in line with the heel of the straightened leg. The untested leg is placed on floor with knee at approximately 90°. At the signal of "Ready! Go!", testee stretch out both arms, palms overlap each other, and reach forward as far as possible at a slow and control motion. Hold about 2 seconds at the maximal reach then relax. Testee should exhale during the reach and inhale during relax. Three trials should be given and the farthest distance is the performance score. Repeat the test with the other leg. Both best-of-three scores are recorded.

Preparation position   Standard posture of the reach</td></tr>
<tr><td rowspan="3">Skinfolds</td><td>Objective</td><td>Assessing body fatness</td></tr>
<tr><td>Equipment</td><td>Skinfold caliper</td></tr>
<tr><td>Instructions</td><td>Skinfold measurement is a good test for estimating percent body fatness. Since specific skills and experience in taking skinfold measurement are required, only trained testers or P.E. teachers are recommended to perform the test. For children and youth, only the triceps and medial calf skinfolds are required. Triceps skinfold site is located at vertical and midway between the acromion process of the scapular and the elbow (see figure below), whereas the medial calf skinfold site is a vertical skinfold taken at the level of maximum circumference of the calf on the right leg (foot rest on a bench so that knee is at 90° angle (see figure below). Each site is measured for at least 2 times and take the average of the two closest values</td></tr>
</table>

(within 2 mm difference). Take the sum of the two skinfold sites and convert to percent fat using the Slaughter et al. (1988) formula.

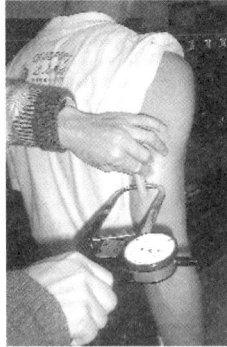

Triceps Skinfold   Medial Calf Skinfold

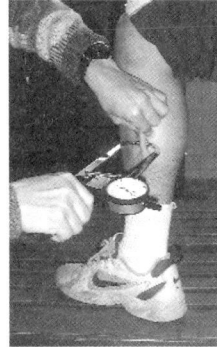

Generalized equation for converting sum of triceps and calf skinfolds to percent fat (Slaughter et al., 1988):

$$\%fat = .610 * (Sum) + [.125 * (Sum) - 4.1] * (gender) + 5.1$$

where Sum is the sum of triceps and calf skinfolds: gender is 1 for boy and 0 for girl.

Appendix 2. Normative Data of the CUHK Health-related Fitness Test

(Reprinted from Hui et al., 2005)

A. Normative Data for Girls

Table 5. Normative data of the One-mile Run (minutes and seconds) for girls (N = 5,303)

Age	Poor (≤16 %tile)	Below Average (17–31 %tile)	Average (32–69 %tile)	Good (70–84 %tile)	Excellent (≥ 85 %tile)
9	≥ 14'19	13'25–14'18	11'36–13'24	10'42–11'35	≤ 10'41
10	≥ 14'54	13'45–14'53	11'27–13'44	10'18–11'26	≤ 10'17
11	≥ 13'27	12'35–13'26	10'50–12'34	09'58–10'49	≤ 09'57
12	≥ 12'50	12'00–12'49	10'21–11'59	09'31–10'20	≤ 09'30
13	≥ 12'24	11'41–12'23	10'16–11'40	09'33–10'15	≤ 09'32
14	≥ 12'25	11'39–12'24	10'07–11'38	09'21–10'06	≤ 09'20
15	≥ 12'31	11'45–12'30	10'13–11'44	09'27–10'12	≤ 09'26
16	≥ 12'24	11'37–12'23	10'03–11'36	09'16–10'02	≤ 09'15
17	≥ 12'12	11'27–12'11	09'57–11'26	09'12–09'56	≤ 09'11
18	≥ 11'48	10'53–11'47	09'03–10'52	08'08–09'02	≤ 08'07
19	≥ 11'39	10'35–11'38	08'26–10'34	07'21–08'25	≤ 07'20

(Adapted from Hui, S.C. (2005). Manual of Health-related Physical Fitness Assessment for Hong Kong Students, Department of Sports Science and Physical Education, The Chinese University of Hong Kong)

Table 6. Normative data of the Modified Push-ups (repetitions) for Girls (N = 5,303)

Age	Poor (≤16 %tile)	Below Average (17–31 %tile)	Average (32–69 %tile)	Good (70–84 %tile)	Excellent (≥ 85 %tile)
9	≤ 1	2–7	8–18	19–23	≥ 24
10	≤ 2	3–7	8–19	20–24	≥ 25
11	≤ 5	6–10	11–19	20–24	≥ 25
12	≤ 6	7–12	13–26	27–32	≥ 33
13	≤ 6	7–14	15–28	29–36	≥ 37
14	≤ 8	9–14	15–27	28–33	≥ 34
15	≤ 7	8–13	14–26	27–32	≥ 33
16	≤ 8	9–13	14–24	25–29	≥ 30
17	≤ 9	10–14	15–24	25–30	≥ 31
18	≤ 10	11–16	17–27	28–33	≥ 34
19	≤ 12	13–18	19–30	31–36	≥ 37

(Adapted from Hui, S.C. (2005). Manual of Health-related Physical Fitness Assessment for Hong Kong Students, Department of Sports Science and Physical Education, The Chinese University of Hong Kong)

Table 7. Normative data of the CUHK Sit-and-reach (cm) Left Leg for girls (N = 5,303)

Age	Poor (≤16 %tile)	Below Average (17–31 %tile)	Average (32–69 %tile)	Good (70–84 %tile)	Excellent (≥ 85 %tile)
9	≤ 45.9	46.0–49.4	49.5–56.4	56.5–59.9	≥ 60.0
10	≤ 44.4	44.5–48.4	48.5–56.4	56.5–60.4	≥ 60.5
11	≤ 44.9	45.0–49.4	49.5–57.4	57.5–61.4	≥ 61.5
12	≤ 47.4	47.5–51.9	52.0–60.9	61.0–64.9	≥ 65.0
13	≤ 48.9	49.0–53.4	53.5–62.4	62.5–66.9	≥ 67.0
14	≤ 49.4	49.5–53.9	54.0–62.9	63.0–67.4	≥ 67.5
15	≤ 48.4	48.5–52.9	53.0–62.9	63.0–67.4	≥ 67.5
16	≤ 48.4	48.5–52.9	53.0–62.4	62.5–66.9	≥ 67.0
17	≤ 48.4	48.5–53.4	53.5–63.4	63.5–68.4	≥ 68.5
18	≤ 48.9	49.0–53.4	53.5–63.4	63.5–68.4	≥ 68.5
19	≤ 41.9	42.0–48.4	48.5–61.9	62.0–68.4	≥ 68.5

(Adapted from Hui, S.C. (2005). Manual of Health-related Physical Fitness Assessment for Hong Kong Students, Department of Sports Science and Physical Education, The Chinese University of Hong Kong)

Table 8. Normative data of the CUHK Sit-and-reach (cm) Right Leg for girls (N = 5,303)

Age	Poor (≤16 %tile)	Below Average (17–31 %tile)	Average (32–69 %tile)	Good (70–84 %tile)	Excellent (≥ 85 %tile)
9	≤ 46.4	46.5–49.9	50.0–57.4	57.5–60.9	≥ 61.0
10	≤ 46.4	45.5–49.4	49.5–56.9	57.0–60.9	≥ 61.0
11	≤ 46.4	46.0–49.9	50.0–57.9	58.0–61.9	≥ 62.0
12	≤ 46.4	48.0–52.4	52.5–61.4	61.5–65.4	≥ 65.5
13	≤ 46.4	49.5–53.9	54.0–62.9	63.0–67.4	≥ 67.5
14	≤ 46.4	49.5–54.4	54.5–63.4	63.5–67.9	≥ 68.0
15	≤ 46.4	49.0–53.4	53.5–62.9	63.0–67.9	≥ 68.0
16	≤ 46.4	49.0–53.4	53.5–62.9	63.0–67.4	≥ 67.5
17	≤ 46.4	49.0–53.9	54.0–63.9	64.0–69.4	≥ 69.5
18	≤ 46.4	49.0–53.9	54.0–63.4	63.5–68.4	≥ 68.5
19	≤ 46.4	43.0–49.9	50.0–62.9	63.0–69.9	≥ 70.0

(Adapted from Hui, S.C. (2005). Manual of Health-related Physical Fitness Assessment for Hong Kong Students, Department of Sports Science and Physical Education, The Chinese University of Hong Kong)

Table 9. Normative data of the Cadence Curl-up (25 reps/min) for girls (N = 5,303)

Age	Poor (≤16 %tile)	Below Average (17–31 %tile)	Average (32–69 %tile)	Good (70–84 %tile)	Excellent (≤ 85 %tile)
9	–	0–3	4–12	13–16	≥ 18
10	≤ 2	3–7	8–16	17–20	≥ 21
11	≤ 4	5–8	9–17	18–22	≥ 23
12	≤ 6	7–12	13–23	24–29	≥ 30
13	≤ 6	7–13	14–28	29–35	≥ 36
14	≤ 8	9–15	16–30	31–37	≥ 38
15	≤ 5	6–13	14–29	30–38	≥ 39
16	≤ 7	8–13	14–27	28–33	≥ 34
17	≤ 7	8–13	14–25	26–31	≥ 32
18	≤ 8	9–14	15–26	27–33	≥ 34
19	≤ 8	9–16	17–31	32–39	≥ 40

(Adapted from Hui, S.C. (2005). Manual of Health-related Physical Fitness Assessment for Hong Kong Students, Department of Sports Science and Physical Education, The Chinese University of Hong Kong)

Table 10. Normative data of Percent Body fat for girls (N = 5,303)

Age	Poor (≤16 %tile)	Below Average (17–31 %tile)	Average (32–69 %tile)	Good (70–84 %tile)	Excellent (≥ 85 %tile)
9	≥ 28	25–27	19–24	16–18	≤ 15
10	≥ 28	25–27	19–24	16–18	≤ 15
11	≥ 28	25–27	19–24	16–18	≤ 15
12	≥ 32	28–31	22–27	18–21	≤ 17
13	≥ 32	29–31	22–28	18–21	≤ 17
14	≥ 34	30–33	23–29	19–22	≤ 18
15	≥ 34	30–33	23–29	20–22	≤ 19
16	≥ 34	30–33	23–29	20–22	≤ 19
17	≥ 33	30–32	23–29	19–22	≤ 18
18	≥ 30	27–29	21–26	18–20	≤ 17
19	≥ 30	26–29	18–25	14–17	≤ 13

(Adapted from Hui, S.C. (2005). Manual of Health-related Physical Fitness Assessment for Hong Kong Students, Department of Sports Science and Physical Education, The Chinese University of Hong Kong)

B. Normative Data for Boys

Table 11. Normative data of the One-mile Run (minutes and seconds) for boys (N = 4,653)

Age	Poor (≤16 %tile)	Below Average (17–31 %tile)	Average (32–69 %tile)	Good (70–84 %tile)	Excellent (≥ 85 %tile)
9	≥ 14'11	13'03–14'10	10'46–13'02	09'28–10'45	≤ 09'27
10	≥ 14'19	12'59–14'18	10'20–12'58	09'00–10'19	≤ 08'59
11	≥ 13'10	12'11–13'09	10'16–12'11	09'18–10'15	≤ 09'17
12	≥ 11'55	10'57–11'54	09'00–10'56	08'02–08'59	≤ 08'01
13	≥ 11'15	10'16–11'13	08'19–10'15	07'20–08'18	≤ 07'19
14	≥ 10'22	09'35–10'21	08'00–09'34	07'12–07'59	≤ 07'11
15	≥ 09'57	09'11–09'56	07'39–09'10	06'53–07'38	≤ 06'52
16	≥ 09'47	09'03–09'46	07'37–09'02	06'54–07'36	≤ 06'53
17	≥ 09'26	08'49–09'25	07'35–08'48	06'58–07'34	≤ 06'57
18	≥ 10'30	09'38–10'29	07'53–09'37	07'01–07'52	≤ 07'00
19	≥ 11'10	10'07–11'09	08'10–10'06	06'59–08'09	≤ 06'58

(Adapted from Hui, S.C. (2005). Manual of Health-related Physical Fitness Assessment for Hong Kong Students, Department of Sports Science and Physical Education, The Chinese University of Hong Kong)

Table 12. Normative data of the Modified Push-up (repetitions) for boys (N = 4,653)

Age	Poor (≤16 %tile)	Below Average (17–31 %tile)	Average (32–69 %tile)	Good (70–84 %tile)	Excellent (≥ 85 %tile)
9	–	0–2	3–9	10–13	≥ 14
10	–	0–2	3–8	9–11	≥ 12
11	–	0–3	4–11	12–15	≥ 16
12	≤ 4	5–9	10–20	21–26	≥ 27
13	≤ 5	6–11	12–22	23–28	≥ 29
14	≤ 8	9–14	15–26	27–31	≥ 32
15	≤ 9	10–16	17–29	30–35	≥ 36
16	≤ 9	10–15	16–28	29–34	≥ 35
17	≤ 11	12–18	19–31	32–38	≥ 39
18	≤ 8	9–15	16–28	29–35	≥ 36
19	≤ 7	8–13	14–27	28–34	≥ 35

(Adapted from Hui, S.C. (2005). Manual of Health-related Physical Fitness Assessment for Hong Kong Students, Department of Sports Science and Physical Education, The Chinese University of Hong Kong)

Table 13. Normative data of the CUHK Sit-and-reach (cm) Left Leg for boys (N = 4,653)

Age	Poor (≤16 %tile)	Below Average (17–31 %tile)	Average (32–69 %tile)	Good (70–84 %tile)	Excellent (≥ 85 %tile)
9	≤ 42.4	42.5–46.4	46.5–53.9	54.0–57.9	≥ 58.0
10	≤ 42.4	42.5–46.4	46.5–53.9	54.0–57.9	≥ 58.0
11	≤ 41.9	42.0–45.9	46.0–53.9	54.0–57.9	≥ 58.0
12	≤ 43.4	43.5–47.4	47.5–55.4	55.5–59.4	≥ 59.5
13	≤ 42.9	43.0–47.4	47.5–56.4	56.5–60.9	≥ 61.0
14	≤ 43.4	43.5–48.4	48.5–57.9	58.0–62.9	≥ 63.0
15	≤ 42.4	42.5–47.4	47.5–58.4	58.5–63.4	≥ 63.5
16	≤ 42.4	42.5–47.9	48.0–58.4	58.5–63.9	≥ 64.0
17	≤ 43.9	44.0–49.4	49.5–60.4	60.5–65.9	≥ 66.5
18	≤ 41.9	42.0–47.4	47.5–58.9	59.0–64.9	≥ 65.0
19	≤ 44.9	45.0–50.4	50.5–61.9	62.0–67.9	≥ 68.

(Adapted from Hui, S.C. (2005). Manual of Health-related Physical Fitness Assessment for Hong Kong Students, Department of Sports Science and Physical Education, The Chinese University of Hong Kong)

Table 14. Normative data of the CUHK Sit-and-reach (cm) Right Leg for boys (N = 4,653)

Age	Poor (≤16 %tile)	Below Average (17–31 %tile)	Average (32–69 %tile)	Good (70–84 %tile)	Excellent (≥ 85 %tile)
9	≤ 47.4	47.5–50.9	51.0–54.4	54.5–57.9	≥ 58.0
10	≤ 46.9	47.0–50.4	50.5–54.4	54.5–57.9	≥ 58.0
11	≤ 46.4	46.5–50.4	50.5–54.4	54.5–58.9	≥ 59.0
12	≤ 48.4	48.5–51.9	52.0–55.9	56.0–59.9	≥ 60.0
13	≤ 47.9	48.0–52.4	52.5–56.9	57.0–61.4	≥ 61.5
14	≤ 48.9	49.0–53.9	54.0–59.4	59.5–64.4	≥ 64.5
15	≤ 48.4	48.5–53.9	54.0–58.9	59.0–64.4	≥ 64.5
16	≤ 48.9	49.0–54.4	54.5–59.9	60.0–64.9	≥ 65.0
17	≤ 49.4	49.5–54.9	55.0–60.4	60.5–66.4	≥ 66.5
18	≤ 48.4	48.5–53.9	54.0–59.4	59.5–65.4	≥ 65.5
19	≤ 51.4	51.5–56.9	57.0–62.9	63.0–68.4	≥ 68.5

(Adapted from Hui, S.C. (2005). Manual of Health-related Physical Fitness Assessment for Hong Kong Students, Department of Sports Science and Physical Education, The Chinese University of Hong Kong)

Table 15. Normative data of Cadence Curl-up (25 reps/min) for boys (N = 4,653)

Age	Poor (≤16 %tile)	Below Average (17–31 %tile)	Average (32–69 %tile)	Good (70–84 %tile)	Excellent (≥ 85 %tile)
9	≤ 1	2–5	6–14	15–18	≥ 19
10	≤ 2	3–6	7–15	16–20	≥ 21
11	≤ 4	5–9	10–19	20–24	≥ 25
12	≤ 7	8–14	15–28	29–34	≥ 35
13	≤ 10	11–17	18–31	32–38	≥ 39
14	≤ 12	13–20	21–36	37–44	≥ 45
15	≤ 14	15–21	22–36	37–44	≥ 45
16	≤ 13	14–20	21–35	36–42	≥ 43
17	≤ 11	12–19	20–35	36–43	≥ 44
18	≤ 6	7–13	14–26	27–33	≥ 34
19	≤ 6	7–13	14–27	28–34	≥ 35

(Adapted from Hui, S.C. (2005). Manual of Health-related Physical Fitness Assessment for Hong Kong Students, Department of Sports Science and Physical Education, The Chinese University of Hong Kong)

Table 16. Normative data of Percent Body fat for boys (N = 4,653)

Age	Poor (≤16 %tile)	Below Average (17–31 %tile)	Average (32–69 %tile)	Good (70–84 %tile)	Excellent (≥ 85 %tile)
9	≥ 29	25–28	16–24	12–15	≤ 11
10	≥ 31	26–30	18–25	13–17	≤ 12
11	≥ 33	28–32	18–27	13–17	≤ 12
12	≥ 31	27–30	17–26	13–16	≤ 12
13	≥ 29	25–28	16–24	12–15	≤ 11
14	≥ 28	24–27	15–23	11–14	≤ 10
15	≥ 26	22–25	14–21	11–13	≤ 10
16	≥ 26	22–25	14–21	10–13	≤ 9
17	≥ 26	22–25	14–21	10–13	≤ 9
18	≥ 28	24–27	16–23	12–15	≤ 11
19	≥ 28	24–27	15–23	11–14	≤ 10

(Adapted from Hui, S.C. (2005). Manual of Health-related Physical Fitness Assessment for Hong Kong Students, Department of Sports Science and Physical Education, The Chinese University of Hong Kong)

PART II

Extent of Physical Activity in Hong Kong Children and Youth

In this section Hong Kong researchers present their findings with regard to the physical activity participation. Employing a variety of the methods discussed in Chapter 2, the authors of the three chapters in Part II describe recent studies (Macfarlane, Chapter 4), summarize series of investigations (Sit, Chow, & Lindner, Chapter 6), and comment on the available literature in this area (McManus, Chapter 5).

Duncan Macfarlane in Chapter 4 reports on a series of three investigations designed to assess physical activity levels in Hong Kong children in primary school grades between 3–6. He uses a subsample of respondents to further examine their activity levels with an habitual physical activity questionnaire, motion monitor and heart rate recording. In a follow-up study, he examines members of the same subsample when they are in high school Forms 1 and 2 with the same techniques. The final study looks at the effects of an intervention programme on activity levels, again with the use of heart rates and motion analysis. Macfarlane's findings are worrying, and he speculates on the possible factors contributing to the low levels of physical activity in his subjects and the lack of effect of intervention.

The focus of Alison McManus in Chapter 5 is on the biological basis of physical activity. Her examination of fitness parameters and their association with activity levels in Hong Kong children shows that there is but little understanding at present of that relationship. She argues against mass fitness testing and the use of age-based norms, and that we are studying the wrong population if we look at Hong Kong children and youth for an understanding of how health-related fitness is linked with being physically active. Establishing norms in an abnormal population is unlikely to benefit this research.

In Chapter 6, Cindy Sit, Ken Chow and Koenraad Lindner report on the physical activity participation data gathered in a series of surveys spanning the past decade, along with participation motives. The high number of respondents who were sedentary confirmed reports presented in the preceding chapters in this section. Data on children with disabilities showed little differences with able-bodied respondents, and that the type of disability was the main determining factor in physical activity participation. Examination of participation motives showed that sport excellence and skill development were not primary reasons for many respondents, but rather fun, fitness and friends. An analysis of contextual factors in intention to participate and actual participation showed the contributions of participants' attitude towards physical activity, parental factors, situational conditions and perceived norms and competence. The chapter closes with a re-examination of the role of physical competence in physical activity participation.

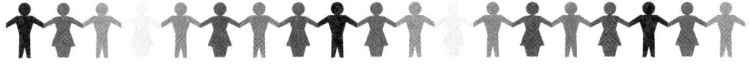

CHAPTER 4

Children's Physical Activity Patterns and the Implications for Health

Duncan Macfarlane

Introduction

This chapter focuses on the results of three complementary studies conducted to first investigate the levels of activity occurring in Hong Kong primary school children and to compare the results with other international studies, thereby providing some "provisional benchmarks" of their physical activity habits; secondly, to examine the degree of tracking in physical activity habits as primary school children move into secondary school; and thirdly, to examine the efficacy of a "Programme for Active Learning" intervention study aimed at increasing physical activity during secondary school hours as well as during discretionary time outside of school. These studies therefore give an overview in Hong Kong of the physical activity habits during primary school, the transition into secondary school, as well as activity patterns in secondary school. Objective measurements of physical activity were performed in all three studies using simultaneous collections of daily heart rates (Polar) and three-dimensional accelerometry (Tritrac), as well as some subjective activity question-naires, in order to provide a degree of comparability across the three studies. Possible contributing factors to the low levels of activity seen in Hong Kong school children and the implications for health are covered in the final sections.

Many public health initiatives aimed at the primary prevention of cardiovascular disease have focused on three major areas, physical activity, dietary cholesterol, and cigarette smoking. The justification is that there is evidence emerging that these habits tend to track into adulthood (Kelder et al., 1994), and it is well known that these areas are primary risk factors associated with the development of chronic degenerative diseases such as Coronary Heart Disease (CHD) in adulthood (Robergs & Roberts, 1997). As Hong Kong has many potential barriers to participation in physical exercise (e.g., climate, pollution, extreme urban density, limited school resources), obtaining detailed objective information on the current levels of activity in its young population will provide important comparative data with other countries. Furthermore, it may provide predictive information on future health risks of its young population.

One underlying assumption in these future predictions is that physical activity habits established during childhood will be carried over into later life. Whether this tracking of physical activity habits occurs is somewhat controversial, as Aaron & Laporte (1997) suggest there is limited evidence to support this notion. However, there is mounting evidence to show there is at least low to moderate levels of tracking of activity from childhood to adulthood (Kelder et al., 1994; Malina, 1996; Telema et al., 1997; Maia et al., 2001). A short summary of recent evidence on the tracking of physical activity by Armstrong & Welsman (1997) concluded that adult exercise patterns may be established during childhood and adolescence, although recent evidence suggests physical inactivity may show a greater degree of tracking. This later view was recently supported by the review of Goran (1998), especially when one considers that a sedentary lifestyle is more important in the development of hypokinetic conditions such as obesity. Thus the information obtained on the activity levels of Hong Kong's young children will allow comparisons of it their current health status with other countries, and provide a possible window into the future health of the territory.

Methods

The data reported here are a summary of some of the results acquired from three studies funded by the Hong Kong Health Services Research Committee that investigated activity levels in primary school, the transition into secondary school, and an intervention study at secondary school.

The first study was in two parts:–

First, it measured the leisure-time energy expenditure from 3,884 Primary 3 to Primary 6 school children (mostly aged 8–11 yr), randomly selected from 30 schools throughout the Hong Kong territory. The instrument used ("CHARG" questionnaire), was a simple self-administered leisure time questionnaire that had previously been found to be acceptably reliable and valid on similar-aged Hong Kong children (Macfarlane & Chan, 1995; Macfarlane, 1997). The CHARG questionnaire categorized both the frequency and duration of 22 common physical activities found in Hong Kong, and together with estimates for intensity taken from a published compendium (Ainsworth et al, 1993), an Activity Metabolic Index (AMI: kJ/kg/d) could be calculated (similar to the AMI that was calculated from the LTPA questionnaire — see below).

Secondly, a sub-sample of 226 of these P3–P6 had their physical activity levels assessed by three methods over one full day:–

(1) the "LTPA" questionnaire was based on the Minnesota Leisure Time Physical Activity (LTPA) questionnaire (Taylor et al., 1978), which is one of the most reliable and valid questionnaires for the measurement of habitual physical activity (Jacobs et al., 1993). The cumulative Activity Metabolic Analysis (AMI) produced by the LTPA questionnaire (i.e., the product of intensity × frequency × duration) is equivalent to an "average energy expenditure" during all physical activities and therefore can be compared with other studies, especially when expressed in units of kJ/kg/d.

(2) at least 10 hours objective monitoring of body movement using a 3-dimensional accelerometer (Tritrac R3D, Hemokinetics, USA) which has been shown to be a valid and reliable measure of physical activity in Hong Kong children (Louie et al., 1999), and has been considered to be superior in assessing children's free play than the uniaxial CSA accelerometer (Ott et al., 2000). The Tritrac data are reported here as the average vector magnitude — "Ave Vect Mag" (counts/min) — the square root of the sum of squares of each of the

three dimensional directions = $(x^2 + y^2 + z^2)^{0.5}$, as has been suggested by McMurray et al (1998), rather than to try to predict energy expenditure using an untested algorithm in children.

(3) at least 10 hours of heart rate recording (PE 4000, Polar Electro, Finland), which is an accepted method for assessing physical activity in children (Freedson & Melanson, 1996; Armstrong & Welsman, 1997). The heart rate data are reported here in two ways: (i) total cumulative time above139 beats/min (an intensity equivalent to low intensity effort); and (ii) total cumulative time above 159 beats/min (an intensity equivalent to moderate intensity effort).

The second study was an attempt to see what happens to activity levels as children moved from primary into secondary school. From the 56 P6 students studied in 1996, 54 were contacted in 1997 when they were in Secondary 1 (S1), but only 36 (67%) gave permission to undergo the same data collection procedures. All 36 students completed the interview-administered Minnesota LTPA questionnaire, but owing to typically unavoidable data collection errors associated with these field measures, only 33 (92%) and 20 (56%) of the students produced analysable 3-D "Tritrac" body motion and heart rate data respectively.

It should be noted in both of these studies that although the monitoring of heart rates and body movement was done in an objective manner, only one single day's recording was made and this may not necessarily reflect the true levels of habitual physical activity for each child. Traditionally at least 2–3 days of monitoring is recommended if one wishes to obtain adequate data to quantify a single individual's levels of habitual activity (Durant et al., 1992; Janz et al, 1995; Trost, 2001; Rowe et al., 2004). However, if the purpose is to report the mean for a sample of the population (as was often the case in the studies reported here), then single-day recordings will provide an adequate measure of the population mean providing adequate samples are taken (as any sampling error will be randomly distributed). The energy expenditures calculated from the subjective questionnaires will, however, provide a reasonable approximation of habitual physical activity, as the subjects were requested to fill these out for a period that covered one full year.

The third study was a 3-month intervention aimed at increasing the levels of habitual physical activity of Hong Kong school children. Two physical education classes involving Form 1 and 2 boys and girls (age 11–13 years) were selected in each of the 10 experimental and 10 control schools. Five students were randomly chosen as target participants from each physical education class, in the experimental and control groups and wore a heart rate monitor (Polar Electro PE4000) and a three-dimensional accelerometer (Tritrac R3D) to simultaneously measure their levels of physical activity over at least 8 continuous hours on two days. Data acquisition began once the student arrived at school and was performed over one school day that included a one-hour physical education class, and one day that did not.

The "Programme for Active Learning" (PAL) intervention focused on three aspects. First, the teachers designed learning experiences that were likely to improve the fitness levels of the participants. The class activities suggested were intended to raise the intensity level of physical activity while teaching sport skills. Second, teachers were asked to set time aside during the class to provide students with the necessary information and encouragement to select activities that they could perform with their parents and siblings so that students would increase their activity at home. This information was included in the guidelines that were distributed to the teachers. Finally, a portfolio was designed and was distributed to students after the pre-test. The primary purpose of the portfolio was to motivate the participants to practice a healthy lifestyle and to form a documented record of involvement (Melograno, 1998).

Results and Discussion

First study: Part 1

A total of 3884 children supplied adequate data for an analysis of the CHARG questionnaire: 45.3% (1748) were girls and 54.7% were boys (2108). Based on the self-reported data collected from the CHARG questionnaire, an "average" Hong Kong primary child claims to exercise on average for about 14–16 minutes, 9–10 times a month, at an intensity of about 5 METs (equivalent to moderate-to-mild exercise). This amount of activity is well below the international recommendations for children (Sallis & Patrick, 1994), and those traditionally cited from the opinion statement produced by the American College of Sports Medicine (1988), on the physical fitness in children and youth. Such recommendations suggest that children should engage in 3 or more activities per week (12 per month) that last at least 20 minutes and require moderate-to-vigorous levels of exertion. Most Hong Kong children do not attain these levels and more than 55% of HK children would be classified as "inactive" and obtain insufficient exercise to promote health-related benefits. This finding is further substantiated from an analysis of the more detailed and objective data on physical activity taken from the sub-sample (see Part 2 below).

First Study: Part 2.

Questionnaire data:
The average AMI value of the Hong Kong primary school children was 10.4 ± 11.8 kJ/kg/d with males producing a significantly greater AMI (13.2 ± 13.3 kJ/kg/d), compared to females (7.5 ± 8.9 kJ/kg/d). To provide an international perspective on these results, a comparison with USA and Canadian data is provided in Table 1.

The review by Blair et al., (1988) suggested that an expenditure of 12.6 kJ/kg/d (3 kcal/kg/d) from physical activity is an acceptable minimum standard in order to accrue significant health-related benefits and to classify the respondent as being "active". Others, such as Riddoch & Boreham (1995) in their review of health-related physical activity in children, also used this value, along with the 1988 Campbell Survey of Well-Being in Canada (Russell et al., 1992). As can be seen from Table 1, only 25% of the children surveyed in Hong Kong were able to meet or exceed this minimum standard, representing 7% of girls and 41% of boys. In comparison, Blair et al. (1988) reported, after re-analysing data on similar aged American children (10–12yr) from the USA National Children and Youth Fitness Survey 1 (NCYFS1, Ross et al., 1985), that 86% of girls and 94% of boys exceeded the standard. Furthermore, data from the Canadian survey on slightly older children (10–14yr), showed that 49% of girls and 72% of boys were classified as being active.

Table 1: Comparison of proportion of girls and boys in the USA, Canada and Hong Kong who met selected leisure-time energy expenditure standards.

	U.S.A. Blair et al '88 age range = 10–12		Canada Stephens & Craig '90 age range = 10–14		Hong Kong '96 Mean age =10.0 range = 8–13	
	Boys n=343	Girls n=235	Boys n=897	Girls n=828	Boys n=118	Girls n=108
Inactive <12.6 kJ/kg/d (<3.0 kcal/kg/d)	6%	14%	28%	51%	59% #	93% #
Active >12.6 kJ/kg/d (>3 kcal/kg/d)	94%	86%	72%	49%	41% #	7% #
Optimally Active >33.6 kJ/kg/d (>8 kcal/kg/d)			40%	33% Data from CFLRI Bull No.13 '97	8% #	2% #

lowest percentage in each category.

In addition, the CFLRI now recommends an AMI of 33.6 kJ/kg/d as being an "optimal" leisure-time energy expenditure for health-related benefits (CFLRI, 1997). They reported that 36% of Canadian children (5–17 yr) reached this standard (40% of boys, 33% of girls), whilst in comparison, a mere 5% of the Hong Kong children reached the same standard (8% of boys, 2% of girls).

It is clear from Table 1 that the Hong Kong children appear considerably less active than their North American counterparts, with a large majority classified as being sedentary, and only a very small percentage are classified as being optimally active. However, some care has to be taken in such comparisons as the samples are not always fully representative of each population (although each sample in Table 1 came from part of a nation-wide survey) and variations in sampling methodology will occur.

(a) Tritrac data:

The average vector magnitude measured in this Hong Kong study was 268.9 ± 87.7 counts/min, with no significant difference found between boys (279.1 ± 90.3) and the girls (258.4 ± 84.1). Unfortunately, comparisons are difficult, as few studies have reported the results from three-dimensional Tritrac accelerometry in free-moving young children using raw Vector Magnitude scores. Many researchers manipulate the raw accelerometry data to predict units of energy expenditure, thereby introducing an unknown error term and this practice has not been recommended on children (McMurray et al, 1998; Crocker et al., 2001); whilst direct comparisons of raw Tritrac scores with other common forms of accelerometry such as the WAM/CSA/MTI accelerometer, are not valid. However, Welk & Corbin (1995) reported the mean value of average vector magnitude across 3 days of monitoring was 482.8 counts/min in 9–11 year old American children, with Coleman et al., (1997) reporting a slightly lower mean of 428.5 counts/min in obese 8–12 year old American children. Quite recent data on slightly younger 6–9 year Australian children (O'Connor et al., 2003) produced a mean of 410 counts/min over a three-day period. Even with these three comparisons, the considerable 35–45% lower values seen in Hong Kong children again demonstrates their comparative lack of habitual physical activity, albeit when compared to a small, non-representative samples of similar-aged American and Australian children.

(b) Heart Rate data:

It has become quite common to report intensity of effort in young children with respect to the amount of time they spend above a specific heart rate thresholds, although again care needs to be taken when interpreting heart rate data from children as many factors can influence their heart rates, especially at lower levels (Armstrong & Welsman, 1997). Heart rate thresholds of 139 and 159 beats/min are quite commonly used as they represent an intensity equivalent to a "brisk walk" and "moderate jog" respectively (Biddle et al., 1991). Several studies have reported the total accumulated time above the 139 and 159 beats/min heart rate thresholds during an average school day using 10–14 hours of recording, with Table 2 providing an international comparison with the Hong Kong data over a similar period.

Table 2: Total Time with Heart Rate above 139 and 159 beats/min in American, Estonian and Singaporean children compared to Hong Kong

	Sallo & Silla '97		Gilbey & Gilbey '95		Simons-Morton et al. '94	Hong Kong '96 Mean age =10.0	
	age range=6–7		age range=9–10		age range = 8–11	range = 8–13	
	(Estonia)		(Singapore)		(America)		
	Boys n=25	Girls n=29	Boys n=50	Girls n=64	Mixed	Boys n=64	Girls n=67
Total time with heart rate above 139 bpm (min)	51	50	47.3	29.6	40.1 n=27 Grade 3 29.2 n=21 Grade 5	27.6 #	27.7 #
Total time with heart rate above 159 bpm (min)	14	12	15.4	10.1	20.0 n=27 Grade 3	8.9 #	7.4 #

lowest percentage in each category.

Some care has to be taken in these comparisons as the samples taken may not have been representative of the population and variations in methodology are likely to occur, such as the length of the measurement period, thus comparisons should only be made over similar lengths of measurement. Although the low sample sizes clearly indicate the studies were not representative, the measurement durations were quite comparable, allowing some tentative comparisons to be made in Table 2. The results again show a tendency that the habitual physical activity levels seen in Hong Kong children are lower than other international studies.

Of particular note is that the Hong Kong children spent less time above both the 139 and 159 beats/min thresholds even when compared to Singaporean children, who have similar urban densities and comparable ethnic, cultural and socio-economic backgrounds to

Hong Kong children, although once again the small sample sizes may not be representative of each population.

Second study (Longitudinal tracking)

Significant tracking of physical activity patterns were seen over the 12 months in both the Tritrac (r=0.41, p<0.034) and LTPA questionnaire data (r=0.52, p<0.001); but significant tracking only occurred in one heart rate variable (activity heart rate; i.e., average heart rate above resting value, (r=0.65, p<0.041). The correlations between variables across the two years were not strong, as were predicted, indicating only a moderate degree of tracking occurred, although they were statistically significant. It was expected that heart rate (and Tritrac) would track (be significantly and positively correlated), but they would not be particularly strong since both measures were taken from only a single 10-hour period. Ideally heart rates and body motion should be studied over a slightly longer period to increase the stability of the measure (Durant et al., 1992; Welk & Corbin, 1995). Since the LTPA questionnaire referred to activities taken over the entire year, it was likely to be more stable and although subjectively acquired, it was likely to be a more reliable indicator of habitual physical activity.

The S1 students showed a significant decrease in overall physical activity levels compared to P6 (MANOVA F=15.82, p=0.011). It can be seen from Table 3 that as Hong Kong Primary-6 children move into Secondary-1 there is a dramatic 46% decrease in their leisure time energy expenditure (LTPA questionnaire). This is a very disconcerting finding, as their P6 activity levels are already very poor, with 60% of the P6 students being classified as "inactive" and less than 9% being classified as "optimally active". Yet within one year of entering secondary school the further reduction in habitual activity meant that now 86% of the S1 cohort was classified as "inactive" and less than 3% being "optimally active". These figures are extremely worrying from a healthcare standpoint. Several possible factors may have contributed to this reduction in activity such as (a) changes from traditionally half-day primary schools to full-day secondary schools, (b) adjustments to a new school environment, and (c) greater academic pressure at secondary schools.

Table 3: Leisure-time energy expenditure of P6 and S1 children and the percentages classified as "inactive" or "optimally active".

	Average LTPA (kJ/kg/d)	Inactive (%) (<12.6 kJ/kg/d)	Optimally Active (%) (>33.6 kJ/kg/d)
Primary-6	14.2	60.0	8.6
Secondary-1	7.7 (46% of P6)	86.2	2.8

Note: "Inactive" = those children with leisure-time energy expenditures less than 12.6 kJ/kg/d and "Optimally active" = those greater than 33.6 kJ/kg/d (CFLRI, 1997).

Table 4: A comparison of the Pre-test and Post-test total time (minutes) spent with Heart Rate above 139 and 159 beats/min on a school day that included a PE lesson for the Control and Experimental students.

	PE lesson day: mean ± S.D. (n: number of subjects)			
	Time (min) > 139 beats.min^{-1}		Time (min) > 159 beats.min^{-1}	
	Pre-test	Post-test	Pre-test	Post-test
Control	43 ± 17 (11)	47 ± 21 (11)	16 ± 10 (11)	18 ± 10 (11)
Experimental	39 ± 28 (20)	41 ± 42 (20)	13 ± 12 (20)	14 ± 21 (20)

Third study (Intervention)

Only those subjects who produced a complete set of analysable pre-test and post-test data (repeated measures data) are shown here and are presented for (a) a day that included a PE lesson, and (b) a non-PE lesson day. However, owing to a variety of logistical, compliance and technical problems with this type of data collection (including two typhoons occurring the post-test phase), the number of successful pairs of pre-test and post-test datasets was markedly lower than expected and it was not possible to re-sample the missing subjects owing to impeding school examinations.

(a) Heart Rate data

As can be seen from the data acquired on a PE lesson day (Table 4), there was considerable consistency across the Control and

Experimental groups over both the pre- and post tests, but with no pre-post test comparisons being statistically significant.

On a day in which no PE lesson occurred, there was a considerable decrease in time spent in above 139 and 159 beats.min^{-1} in the post-test results (Table 5), yet none of these changes were statistically significant either.

Table 5: **A comparison of the Pre-test and Post-test total time (minutes) spent with Heart Rate above 139 and 159 beats/min on a school day that did not include a PE lesson for the Control and Experimental students.**

	Non-PE lesson day: mean ± S.D. (n: number of subjects)			
	Time (min) > 139 beats.min^{-1}		Time (min) > 159 beats.min^{-1}	
	Pre-test	Post-test	Pre-test	Post-test
Control	12 ± 12 (6)	4 ± 3 (6)	3 ± 5 (36)	2 ± 2 (12)
Experimental	23 ± 33 (17)	18 ± 30 (17)	10 ± 12 (17)	5 ± 12 (17)

(b) Tritrac data.

When the Tritrac Average Vector Magnitude data were analysed (Table 6) there was a slight trend towards the Experimental group producing change scores that were larger than the Control group (a 0% decrease in the Experimental group on the Non-PE day compared to a 6.8% decrease in the Control group; a 7.2% decrease in the Control PE group, compared to a 1.6% increase in the Experimental group), none of these changes were statistically significant.

Overall, the heart rate and Tritrac body movement monitoring showed the Experimental group had generally no significant improvement in their activity patterns as a result of the intervention. This lack of an intervention effect was seen in both the PE lesson, where, if anything, a positive effect was to be expected, and also in the whole day data, which failed to show any effect on discretionary activity patterns. Although some small positive trends were seen in some variables in the Experimental group when compared to the Control group, the effects were not very encouraging. One possible reason for the decline in activity patterns seen on the Post-test, especially on

Table 6: A comparison of the Pre-test and Post-test Average Vector Magnitude data (counts/minutes) on a school day that did and did not include a PE lesson for the Control and Experimental students.

	Average Vector Magnitude (counts.min⁻¹) mean ± S.D. (n: number of subject)			
	Non-PE lesson day		PE lesson day	
	Pre-test	Post-test	Pre-test	Post-test
Control	217 ± 70 (26)	202 ± 83 (26)	320 ± 115 (24)	297 ± 98 (24)
Experimental	217 ± 123 (61)	217 ± 85 (61)	268 ± 103 (53)	273 ± 95 (53)

Non-PE days in Table 5, was that the students were preparing for the forthcoming exams, for which there is considerable pressure to succeed (Johns & Dimmock, 1999). As a result, these students are likely to have reduced their discretionary physical activities in favour of studying. It is also possible that the students were either resistance to the PAL intervention, or that this type of intervention was not as practical for busy teachers to implement (Johns et al, 2001).

Are Hong Kong children the most inactive?

There is quite reasonable and consistent evidence to support the notion that Hong Kong children are probably the most inactive students in the world, based on current comparisons from the sports science literature. The data used to reach this conclusion are not taken from one study, nor from only one assessment technique, but involve several studies using a mixture of both subjective data from activity questionnaires as well as objective measures taken from both heart rate monitors and 3-dimensional accelerometers. Although only parts of the results of the above studies have been presented here, when all the data were used, a total of 28 "physical activity variables" on Hong Kong children were compared across 16 different international studies. Although direct comparisons with other studies have many limitations and only when identical measures are used simultaneously across international studies (e.g., using the International Physical Activity Questionnaire — IPAQ; Craig et al., 2003; Brown et al., 2004), can true comparisons be made with confidence, it was disconcerting to find that Hong Kong students ranked the lowest, in 23 of the 28 comparisons, and were second-lowest in the remaining 5 comparisons. In spite of the limitations of these types of comparisons, a reasonably clear trend emerges from these studies using a number of measurement techniques that suggests quite strongly that, according to current published literature, Hong Kong children are likely candidates to be the most physically inactive students in the world.

It is likely that other children may face similar barriers to physical activity, such as in other territories with extreme urban densities (e.g., Japan or Macau), yet there is not sufficient data available to show how students in these areas compare with Hong Kong students. Thus until other evidence emerges, it can be tentatively concluded that Hong Kong children are likely to have the unfortunate mantle of being the most inactive students in the published literature.

Possible contributing factors to low activity levels in Hong Kong children.

Many factors may contribute to the barriers faced by Hong Kong children. A number of these potential barriers are listed below, many of which are speculative and are open to conjecture. Yet when combined together, they provide a rather unique set of circumstances that may explain why Hong Kong's young children have become very inactive.

A) Environment:

Lack of opportunities: Hong Kong has a high population density (eg., Kwun Tong district has 54,620 people/square km; Howlett, 1999), most families living in small high-rise apartments with a gross floor areas normally much less than 1,000 square feet. Hong Kong also has a highly congested road network (averaging 268 vehicles per kilometre of road: Howlett, 1999), thus opportunities for free-play at home or cycling/playing on the street are extremely limited.

Climate: Being a typically semi-tropical climate, the hot and humid Hong Kong environment can provide a strong disincentive to perform exercise.

Highly efficient public transport: The tremendous availability of frequent and cheap public transport reduces the need to walk any significant distance. In addition, elevators and escalators have made stair-climbing almost an unnecessary act.

B) Society:

Concept of health: Perhaps then notion of health in Hong Kong is becoming viewed more as an absence of disease, rather than a state of good physical condition that requires regular physical exercise.

Working parents: It is common for both parents to work in Hong Kong, thus leaving children in the care of other care-givers such as grandparents or domestic helpers, who may not provide physically active role models.

Academic pressures: Parents, and educators, in Hong Kong have always placed great emphasis on their children's academic education, however, this may be to the detriment of their child's physical activity habits (Johns & Ha, 1999).

C) Central Administration:

Resources: Schools seem to lack the space and facilities needed to run effective curricula and extra-curricula activity programmes, with nearly 50% of primary school PE teachers feeling their equipment and facilities were below the Education Department standards (To, 1985).

Education Department: Perhaps more pressure could have been exerted by the Education Department to introduce reforms earlier (e.g., more PE classes in the curriculum, more full-day schools, less focus on examinations, more activities that are enjoyable and serve as foundations for future participation). The Curriculum Development Council of the Hong Kong Education Department has responded in many ways to these needs and in 2002 released a Key Learning Area (KLA) curriculum guide specifically for Physical Education that addresses some of these issues.

D) Schools:

Status of PE: Physical education classes generally suffer from a low status and are viewed as a low-priority programme (Johns & Dimmock, 1999).

Resources: Many PE teachers feel that their school principals do not provide adequate financial or moral support for their PE programmes. Furthermore, few primary schools have and indoor gymnasium and must often rely on one outdoor basketball court for most PE activities (Fu, 1988).

Problems with PE lessons: A recent study (Macfarlane & Wong,

2003) has shown that Hong Kong Primary school children do not receive sufficient physical activity in the PE lessons to achieve some recommended international guidelines. A normal Hong Kong PE class only used 22 of the 35-minute class time, with students averaging less than 4 minutes of moderate-to-vigorous activity and most PE activities receiving a low enjoyment rating.

Inappropriate activities: There may be some tendency for schools to focus excessively on activities that are associated with inter-school competitions, which may be detrimental to more esoteric and individual sports, or those likely to serve as a foundation for activities in later life.

Conclusions

It has become clear that, for a combination of possibly unique reasons, young Hong Kong school children have adopted very sedentary lifestyles and are either resistant to interventions aimed at improving these levels or that more effective interventions need to be trialled. The amount of activity these students acquire does not come close to reaching the levels currently recommended by international authorities for the development and maintenance of good health either during the day or in their PE lessons. Furthermore, even though the data presented here may not represent the true levels of habitual physical activity (see caveat earlier due to a single-day recording), the Hong Kong children would appear to be candidates for having the lowest levels of physical activity cited in the academic literature to date. It is particularly concerning when this level of physical inactivity is combined with the knowledge that Hong Kong's children (i) have high levels of blood cholesterol (Leung, 1995), (ii) are exposed to unhealthy levels of environmental tobacco smoke (Lam et al., 1998; Lam et al., 1999), and (iii) have rising levels of obesity (Leung et al., 1998). All of these factors are primary and modifiable risk factors for CHD. It is clear that Hong Kong's administrators, parents, teachers and health professionals all need to recognise the magnitude of this problem and react constructively to it, else Hong Kong's children are likely to incur significant and costly medical problems in the near future (Adab & Macfarlane, 1998).

Acknowledgements

The results presented here were from a series of research projects funded by the Hong Kong Health Services Research Committee.

References

Aaron, D. J., & Laporte, R. E. (1997). Physical activity, adolescence, and health: an epidemiological perspective. *Exercise and Sports Science Reviews, 25*, 391–405.

Adab, P., & Macfarlane, D. J. (1998). Exercise and health — new imperatives for public health policy in Hong Kong. *Hong Kong Medical Journal, 4*, 389–393.

Ainsworth, B. E., Haskell, W. L., Leon, A. S., Jacobs, D. S., Montoye, H. L., Sallis, J. F., & Paffenbarger, R. S. (1993). Compendium of physical activities: classification of energy costs of human physical activities. *Medicine and Science in Sports and Exercise, 25*, 71–80.

American College of Sports Medicine (1988). Opinion statement on physical fitness in children and youth. *Medicine and Science in Sports and Exercise, 20*, 422–423.

Armstrong, N. & Welsman, J. (1997). *Young people and physical activity.* Oxford: Oxford University Press.

Biddle, S., Mitchell, J., & Armstrong, N. (1991). The assessment of physical activity in children: a comparison of continuous heart rate monitoring, self-report, and interview recall techniques. *British Journal of Physical Education, 10*(suppl.), 5–8

Blair, S. N., Clark, D. G., Cureton, K. J., & Powell, K. E. (1988). Exercise and fitness in childhood: Implications for a lifetime of health. In D. R. Lamb & C. V. Gisolfi. (Eds.), *Perspectives in Exercise Science and Sports Medicine, Vol. 2: Youth Exercise and Sport,* Carmel, Indiana: Benchmark.

Brown, W. J., Trost, S. G., Bauman, A., Mummery, K. & Owen, N. (2004). Test-retest reliability of four physical activity measures used in population surveys. *Journal of Science and Medicine in Sport, 7*, 205–215.

CFLRI — Canadian Fitness and Lifestyle Research Institute (1997). *Bulletin 13,* Canada: CFLRI.

Coleman, K. J., Saelens, B. E., Wiedrich-Smith, M. D., Finn, J. D., & Epstein, L. H. (1997). Relationship between Tritrac-R3D vectors, heart rate, and self-report in obese children. *Medicine and Science in Sports and Exercise,* 29, 1535–1542.

Craig, C. L., Marshall, A. L., Sjostrom, M., Bauman, A. E., Booth, M. L., Ainsworth, B. E., Pratt, M., Ekelund, U., Yngve, A., Sallis, J. F., & Oja, P. (2003). International physical activity questionnaire: 12-country reliability and validity. *Medicine and Science in Sports and Exercise,* 35, 1381–1395.

Crocker, P. R. E., Holowachuk, D. R. & Kowalski, K. C. (2001). Freasibility of using the Tritrac motion sensor over a 7-day trial with older children. *Pediatric Exercise Science,* 13, 70–81.

Durant, R.H., Baranowski, T., Davis, H., Thompson, W. O., Puhl, J., Greaves, K. A., & Rhodes, T. (1992). Reliability and variability of heart rate monitoring in 3-, 4- or 5-yr-old children. *Medicine and Science in Sports and Exercise,* 24, 265–271.

Freedson, P. S., & Melanson, E. L. (1996). Measuring physical activity. In D. Docherty (Ed.) *Measurement in Pediatric Exercise Science* (pp. 261–283). Champaign: Human Kinetics.

Fu, F. H. (1988). School Physical Education in Hong Kong. *Physical Education Review,* 11, 147–152.

Gilbey, H., & Gilbey, M. (1995). The physical activity of Singapore primary school children as estimated by heart rate monitoring. Pediatric Exercise Science, 7, 26–35.

Goran, M. I. (1998). Measurement issues related to studies of childhood obesity: assessment of body composition, body fat distribution, physical activity, and food intake. *Pediatrics,* (suppl.) 101, 505–518.

Howlett, B (ed), (1999). *Hong Kong 1998.* Hong Kong: Information Services Department.

Jacobs, D. R., Ainsworth, B. E., Hartman, T. J., & Leon, A. S. (1993). A simultaneous evaluation of 10 commonly used physical activity question-naires. *Medicine and Science in Sports and Exercise,* 25, 81–91.

Janz, K. F., Witt, J. & Mahoney, L. T. (1995). The stability of children's physical activity as measured by accelerometry and self-report. *Medicine and Science in Sports and Exercise,* 27, 1326–1332.

Johns, D. P., & Dimmock, C. (1999). The marginalization of physical education: impoverished curriculum policy and practice in Hong Kong. *Journal of Education Policy, 14,* 363–384.

Johns, D. P., & A. S. Ha. (1999). Home and recess physical activity of Hong Kong Children. *Research Quarterly for Exercise and Sport,* 70, 319–323.

Johns, D. P., Ha, A. S. C, & Macfarlane, D. J. (2001). Raising activity levels: a multi-dimensional analysis of curriculum change. *Sport Education and Society*, 6, 199–210.

Kelder, S. H., Perry, C. L., Klepp, K-I., & Lytle, L. L. (1994). Longitudinal tracking of adolescent smoking, physical activity, and food choice behaviours. *American Journal of Public Health*, 84, 1121–1126.

Lam, T. H., Chung, S. F., Betson, C. L., Wong, C. M., & Hedley, A. J. (1998). Respiratory symptoms due to active and passive smoking in junior secondary school students in Hong Kong. *International Journal of Epidemiology*, 27, 41–48.

Lam, T. H., Hedley, A. J., Chung, S. F., & Macfarlane, D. J. (1999). Passive smoking and respiratory symptoms in primary school children in Hong Kong. *Human and Experimental Toxicology*, 18, 218–223.

Leung, S. S. F. (1995). Childhood obesity in Hong Kong. *Hong Kong Journal of Paediatrics*, 1 (suppl), 63–68.

Leung, S. S. F., Chan, Y. L., Lam, C. W. K., Peng, X. H., Woo, K. S. & Metreweli, C. (1998). Body fatness and serum lipids of 11-year-old Chinese children. *Acta Paediatrica*, 87, 363–367.

Louie, L., Eston, R. G., Rowlands, A. N., Tong, K. K., Ingledew, K., & Fu, F. H. (1999). Validity of heart rate, pedometry, and accelerometry for estimating energy cost of activity in Hong Kong Chinese boys. *Pediatric Exercise Science*, 11, 229–239.

Macfarlane, D. J., & Chan, M. K. (1995, November). *Reliability of a questionnaire to investigate differences in habitual physical activity of Hong Kong primary school children — a pilot study.* Paper presented at the conference on Gender Issues in Sport and Exercise, Hong Kong Sport Development Board, Hong Kong.

Macfarlane, D. J., & Wong, T. K. (2003). Children's heart rates and enjoyment levels during PE classes in Hong Kong primary schools. *Pediatric Exercise Science*, 15, 179–190.

Macfarlane, D. J. (1997, March). *Examining the validity of a self-administered questionnaire to investigate the habitual physical activity of Hong Kong primary school children.* Paper presented at the conference on Health, Physical Activity and Children in Hong Kong, University of Hong Kong, Hong Kong.

Maia, J. A. R., Lefevre, J., Claessens, A., Renson, R., Vanreusel, B., & Beunen, G. (2001). Tracking of physical fitness during adolescence: a panel study in boys. *Medicine and Science in Sports and Exercise*, 33, 765–771.

Malina, R. M. (1996). Tracking of physical activity and physical fitness across the lifespan. *Research Quarterly for Exercise and Sport, 67,* 48–57.

McMurray, R. G., Harrell, J. S., Bradley, C. B., Webb, J. P. & Goodman, E. M. (1998). Comparison of a computerized physical activity recall with a triaxial motion sensor in middle-school youth. *Medicine and Science in Sports and Exercise, 30,* 1238–1245.

Melograno, V. (1998). *Professional and student portfolios for physical education.* Champaign, IL: Human Kinetics.

O'Connor, J., Ball, E. J., Steinbeck, K. S., Davies, P. S. W., Wishart, C., Gaskin, K. J. & Baur, L. A. (2003). Measuring physical activity in children: a comparison of four different methods. *Pediatric Exercise Science, 15,* 202–215.

Ott, A. E., Pate, R. R., Trost, S. G., Ward, D. S. & Saunders, R. (2000). The use of uniaxial and triaxial accelerometers to measure children's "free-play" physical activity. *Pediatric Exercise Science, 12,* 360–370.

Riddoch, C. J., & Boreham, C. A. G. (1995). The health-related physical activity of children. *Sports Medicine, 19,* 86–102.

Roberts, R. A., & Roberts, S. O. (1997). *Exercise Physiology: exercise, performance, and clinical applications.* St Louis: Mosby.

Ross, J. G., Dotson, C. O. & Gilbert, G. G. (1985). Are kids getting appropriate activity? *Journal of Physical Education, Recreation and Dance, 56,* 82–85.

Rowe, D. A., Mahar, M. T., Raedeke, T. D. & Lore, J. (2004). Measuring physical activity in children with pedometers: reliability, reactivity, and replacement of missing data. *Pediatric Exercise Science, 16,* 343–354.

Russell, S. J., Hyndford, C., & Beaulieu, A. (1992). *Active living for Canadian children and youth: A statistical profile.* Ottawa: Canadian Fitness and Lifestyle Research Institute.

Sallis, J. F., & Patrick, K. (1994). Physical activity guidelines for adolescents: Consensus statement. *Pediatriac Exercise Science, 6,* 302–314.

Sallo, M., & Silla, R. (1997). Physical activity with moderate to vigorous intensity in preschool and first-grade schoolchildren. *Pediatric Exercise Science, 9,* 44–54.

Simons-Morton, B. G., Taylor, W. C., & Huang, I. W. (1994). Validity of the Physical Activity Interview and Caltrac with preadolescent children. *Research Quarterly for Exercise and Sport, 65,* 84–88.

Stephens, T. & Craig, C. L. (1990). *The well-being of Canadians: The 1988 Campbell's survey.* Ottawa: Canadian Fitness and Lifestyle Research Institute.

Taylor, H. L., Jacobs, D.R., Schucker, B., Knudsen, J., Leon, A.S., & Debacker, G. (1978). A questionnaire for the assessment of leisure time physical activities. *Journal of Chronic Disease*, 31, 741–755.

Telema, R., Yang, X., Laakso, L., Viikari, J. (1997). Physical activity in childhood as predictor of physical activity in young adulthood. *American Journal of Preventive Medicine*, 13, 317–323.

To, C. Y. (1985). *Physical Fitness of Children in Hong Kong*. Hong Kong: Chinese University of Hong Kong,

Trost, S. G. (2001). Objective measurement of physical activity in youth: Current issues, future directions. *Exercise and Sports Science Review*, 29, 32–36.

Welk, G. J., & Corbin, C. B. (1995). The validity of the Tritrac-R3D activity monitor for the assessment of physical activity in children. *Research Quarterly for Exercise and Sport*, 66, 202–209.

CHAPTER *5*

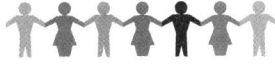

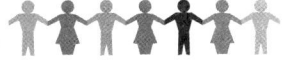

Health-related Physical Activity Habits of Hong Kong Youth

Ali McManus

Introduction

For many it is a remarkable paradox that when the most rigorous measures are used, only a meagre, or no relationship is observed between physical activity and aspects of health-related functioning in children. Perhaps this is simply an outcome of those being assessed. The typical activity bouts characterizing the majority of the participants in the available studies of Hong Kong youth would result in physiological effort of not even moderate intensity. One could argue that if we want to understand the determinants of being a physically active child, we need to study physically active children.

Understanding the health-related outcomes of physical activity in youngsters requires acknowledgement that the exact nature of physical activity is complex and an intricate combination of both the biological and behavioural. Most of the research attention in Hong Kong has focused on characterising physical activity patterns, and upon understanding the behavioural component of activity, such as the motivation for activity participation or the potential influence of the social and physical environments, such as the home or school. Much less attention has focused on understanding the biological basis of physical activity.

The biological purpose of physical activity is most likely related to motor and neural development in the child, which, in the absence of physical activity may result in reduced appropriate motor experiences, ultimately limiting the differentiation of active behaviour. This chapter begins by exploring aspects of health-related fitness (with the exception of body composition which is dealt with in chapters 7 and 8), in Chinese youngsters, and finishes by discussing the potential biological precursors of physical activity habits in children.

The role physical activity plays in maintaining health and preventing lifestyle related disease is now well established. Recent data from China show that lifetime physical activity can reduce the risk for breast cancer (Matthews, Shu, Jin, et al., 2001), and improve lipid profiles (Hu, Pekkarinen, Hanninen, et al., 2002). Heart disease is now the second major cause of death in Hong Kong. It has been estimated that 42% of men have a 1 in 5 chance of developing coronary heart disease and 48% of women have a 1 in 10 chance of developing coronary heart disease (Chan, Chu, Ko, et al., 1999). This is significant when we consider that approximately 20% of Hong Kong children are obese (Leung, Chan, Lam, et al., 1998), and blood lipid profiles in Hong Kong children are so elevated that they are amongst the highest in the world (Leung et al., 1998). The degree to which increasing levels of physical activity can prevent poor health outcomes in childhood has been the topic of much research. Results however, are inconsistent and conflict within the literature makes it difficult to draw any definitive conclusions.

Reliable physical activity data for Chinese youngsters have been available for a number of decades. The earliest of these studies (Banerjee & Saha, 1982) characterised the energy cost of common physical activities in 12–14 year old Chinese boys in Singapore using respiratory gas analysis. In 1999, a similar study was conducted (Louie, Eston, Rowlands, et al., 1999) with 8–10 year-old Chinese boys in Hong Kong. Both studies showed that activities such as writing or crayoning cost minimal energy. In contrast running costs approximately five-times more energy than writing or crayoning.

Later work has focused largely upon characterizing the physical activity habits of Hong Kong youth. Of the various published studies, utilising a range of methodologies (*heart rate telemetry*: Barnett, Bacon-Shone, Tam, Leung, & Armstrong, 1995; McManus & Armstrong,

1996a; Wong, 1997; *motion analysis*: Louie et al., 1999; Macfarlane, 1997; Rowlands, Eston, Louie, et al., 2002; *participant observation*: Johns & Ha, 1999; *questionnaire*: Lindner, 1998; Macfarlane, 1997; Ng, 1996), all have concluded that few Hong Kong children achieve the levels of physical activity associated with the improvement or maintenance of aerobic fitness.

Wong's (1997) work highlighted that over a ten hour monitoring period, Hong Kong Chinese primary school children spent only 3.8% of their time engaged in moderate level physical activity (heart rate $\geq$ 139 beats per minute). In contrast, it is recommended that children accumulate at least one hour of moderate intensity activity on most days of the week (Haennel & Lemire, 2002). Low levels of physical activity have been found to be particularly problematic in girls. McManus & Armstrong (1996a) indicated that none of the 8–9 year-old Hong Kong Chinese girls they monitored over three days experienced a single ten minute period with heart rate above 159 beats per minute (equivalent to slow jogging). Only one percent achieved a five-minute bout of activity in this heart rate zone.

Louie et al.'s (1999) paper makes a very important contribution to our interpretation of motion analysis physical activity data for Chinese children, because the energy cost of various activities, such as writing, playing hopscotch, walking and running, are translated into triaxial accelerometer (Tritrac) counts per minute, as well as pedometer counts per minute.

Similarly low levels of physical activity have been recorded in other Chinese populations. Singaporean Chinese children demonstrated low levels of physical activity, with girls less active than boys (Gilbey & Gilbey, 1995; Schmidt, Stensel, & Walkuski, 1997). Marked differences in physical activity levels between Asian* and Caucasian pubescent girls residing in Canada have also been identified (Mackelvie, Mckay, Khan, & Crocker, 2001). The Caucasian girls in this study engaged in

---

* It should be noted that whilst the majority of the Asian children in the two studies from Canada (Mackelvie et al., 2001, and McKay et al. 2000) were Chinese, the Asian subjects also included children with parents from the Phillipines, Japan and Vietnam.

almost twice the amount of physical activity compared to the Asian girls, with 5.9 hours per week of physical activity at an intensity greater than walking being recorded in the Caucasian girls compared to only 3.3 hours per week in the Asian girls. Another study from the same Canadian group (McKay, Petit, Khan, & Schutz, 2000), working with 8-9 year old boys and girls notes a rather different pattern, with Asian girls 8% more physically active than Asian boys. Although a number of published studies now exist which describe the volume and intensity of physical activity levels by age or by sex, the influence of culture and context on these patterns has been largely neglected in the Asian population.

It is clear that Hong Kong youngsters are physically inactive. The extent to which this sedentary lifestyle affects aspects of health-related function is however far less clear. To date no study has systematically examined the relationship between objectively assessed physical activity, and gold standard measures of the various components of health-related fitness. Understanding the possible influence of sedentarianism in our young population may instead be gained by considering those data that describe aspects of health-related fitness in comparison, where appropriate, with values from more active populations. The use of field test batteries of health- related fitness components has been prolific in Hong Kong school students and this means there is a fairly abundant source of cross-sectional data on health-related physical performance across various age groups in Chinese youth (Hatano, Hua, Jiang, et al., 1997; Eston, Ingledew, Fu, & Rowlands, 1998). No published Hong Kong study and only a few with mainland Chinese youngsters have compared performance in a range of field fitness test by both age and maturational stage (Ji, 2001; Ohsawa, Ji, & Kasai, 1997). This is disappointing given how important biological maturation is in the interpretation of performance measures, measures that are far more dependent on maturational age than chronological age (Matsudo, 1996). Comparisons of data therefore between Hong Kong girls and boys and Chinese children from elsewhere in China or Caucasian children should be made cautiously, because of the advanced maturational timing of southern and urban Chinese, compared to northern or rural Chinese or Caucasians.

Aerobic Fitness

Documented accounts of laboratory assessed aerobic fitness in Hong Kong children and adolescents, although limited, are available. Barnett et al. (1995) and McManus & Armstrong (1996b) found similar values for 12–16 year olds, values that are fairly consistent with other studies for Caucasian adolescents within this age range (Eisenmann & Malina, 2002). The data published by Tong et al. (2001), for 17 year-olds, are considerably higher than either those of Barnett et al. (1995) or McManus and Armstrong (1996b). Peak oxygen uptake values for American male and female 16 year-olds in the 1990s were reported by Eisenmann & Malina (2002) as 45.6 and 33.4 ml.kg^{-1}min^{-1} respectively, much lower than the values reported by Tong, Fu, & Chow (2001), particularly when one considers that 31 of Tong et al.'s 45 subjects were females.

Published data for younger Hong Kong children are less consistent. Data from McManus, Hung and Tung (2002) found values 75% lower than expected age norms generated from the regression equations of Armstrong, Welsman, & Kirby (2000). In contrast, Chan and Hui (2000) found peak VO$_2$ to be 46.6 and 50.0 ml.kg^{-1}min^{-1} in 8 to 12 year old girls and boys respectively. Chan and Hui's data fit exactly with the age norm calculated from Armstrong & Welsman's (2000) regression equation, and are nearly identical to values for similarly aged British children (Armstrong, Kirby, McManus & Welsman, 1995). A more detailed account of the peak VO$_2$ of Hong Kong Chinese youngsters by age, maturity and sex is needed before any accurate profile of what constitutes 'normal' can be generated, and any association between physical activity and aerobic fitness remains inconclusive.

Numerous field tests exist which predict peak VO$_2$ from either submaximal or maximal data. The most popular of these is probably the multi-stage shuttle run. A number of studies with Hong Kong youngsters have been published utilizing this method. The first of these was from Barnett, Chan, and Bruce (1993) in adolescent girls and boys. More recently data published by Wong, Yu, Wang, & Robinson (2001) estimated peak VO$_2$ using the 20-m shuttle run in 8–12 year olds. Wong et al.'s boys and girls reached a mean exercise level equivalent to a running speed of 10 to 10.5 km.h^{-1}, whilst Barnett's subjects attained maximal running speeds of 11 to 11.7 km.h^{-1}. The difference in speed is probably quite simply a reflection of size, however, the difference in the peak VO$_2$ values predicted from the two data sets is quite striking. Wong et al. (2001) report very low values for their subjects (boys: 30.3±5.2; girls: 28.6±3.6) in comparison to Barnett et al. (1993). Such differences in predicted VO$_2$ may be accounted for by the different prediction equations used by these authors. It should also be remembered that the shuttle run was developed with Caucasian adults and the speeds may be inappropriately fast. With no ability to increase intensity beyond maximal running speed, caution must be exerted when interpreting results from these field estimates since low levels may reflect test inadequacy rather than physical inactivity.

Physical activity guidelines for children initially placed emphasis on sustained periods of moderate to vigorous physical activity (Sallis & Patrick, 1994). This may account for the preoccupation with finding a relationship between physical activity and prolonged maximal aerobic power output. Paradoxically, when the most rigorous measures are used, only a meagre, or no relationship has been observed between physical activity and aerobic fitness in studies of Caucasian children. Perhaps this is not unsurprising when one considers that children are essentially anaerobic movers. As Åstrand noted in 1952 (cited in Van Praagh, 2000, p. 150),

> *Children … readily strain themselves maximally for some seconds but heartily dislike monotonous, heavy work. Their way of living is rather of an "anaerobic" character.*

This classic spontaneity has been substantiated by the very elegant analyses provided by Berman et al. (1998). These analyses show the physical activity patterns of prepubertal children to be frequent (26–28 bouts per hour), variable in intensity, and of short duration (20–21 seconds per bout). More in keeping with the characteristic spontaneity of childhood activity patterns, physical activity guidelines have recently shifted towards accumulating activity over a day rather than focusing on sustained periods of physical activity (National Institutes of Health, 1996). However, the evidence that health benefits may be gained from accumulating activity in short bouts over a day has been challenged (Hardman, 1999).

Even benefits to aerobic fitness from sustained exercise have been varied in children. To date, only one published study is available which documents change in aerobic fitness in Hong Kong Chinese youngsters. Cheng, McManus, & Macfarlane (2002) found no significant changes in peak VO_2 following eight weeks of training on cycle ergometers, three times per week for 20 minutes per session. Intensity was monitored in these boys using heart rate telemetry, and was maintained at 60–70% maximum heart rate. Given aerobic fitness has a relatively large genetic component, should we even expect physical activity to directly relate to aerobic fitness values in low-active children?

Muscular Strength and Endurance

There is a similar paucity of data on the development of muscular strength from childhood through the maturational period. Field tests of muscular endurance (sit-ups, pull-ups) and muscular strength (grip strength) have been published in various reports, the most recent of which is from the Macau Education and Youth Department (2000). Similar to European data (Beunen, Ostyn, Simons, et al., 1997) static strength, assessed using a hand grip dynamometer, increased fairly linearly in Chinese boys from Macau, with a marked acceleration at approximately 12–13 years. In the Chinese girls from Macau, grip strength also increased linearly, but without a dramatic adolescent spurt. Evidence from studies elsewhere suggest that the adolescent spurt in strength development usually begins before the peak height velocity by about one to one and a half years. During this peak strength development period boys will gain approximately 30% of their eventual peak strength.

The developmental pattern of functional strength (muscular endurance) assessed by number of sit-ups in a given time also increases with age. Data from Macau are nearly identical to those published on Flemish boys and girls in the 1980s (Beunen et al., 1988) with a similar decline in girls noticeable for both populations at approximately 13 years of age. Peak strength of girls is about half that of boys. Peak strength and muscular endurance differ little from data for Caucasian children collated over the past 20 years. It is unlikely that we can draw any conclusions regarding the role sedentarianism may be playing in developmental patterns of peak strength and muscular endurance in Chinese children.

Flexibility

Hatano et al. (1997) published sit and reach values for Chinese children aged 10 to 17 years from Shanghai, Macau and Hong Kong. The Shanghai girls and boys had consistently higher values, whilst the two southern Chinese groups (Macau and Hong Kong) recorded remarkably similar values by age and sex. Despite the authors' conclusion that these differences between the Shanghainese children and Southern Chinese were a marker of the increased fitness of the Shanghai population, it is more likely that they are simply a reflection of the lager body size of the more northerly Chinese.

Understanding physical activity behaviour

Primary school physical education is arguably the most important time for fostering in children an appreciation for being physically active yet even the Government of Hong Kong (2002) in its most recent consultative document, *The Sports Policy Review* acknowledged that current physical education has failed to foster these habits. At both primary and secondary levels, the health and physical activity message has been delivered via battery fitness testing which has been shown to be less than successful in promoting the advantages of physical activity, especially for girls. Mass fitness testing in schools use norm tables for the local population constructed on the basis of age rather than maturity and they also provide different norms for girls and boys. This difference in expectation has been felt to further exacerbate the problem with girls since it encourages teachers to accept lower norms for girls as reflecting acceptable performances, such that girls then tend to meet these lower expectations.

Given the documented low levels of physical activity, but the seemingly marginal impact these are having on traditionally assessed aspects of health-related fitness, the question of whether we are focusing on the wrong parameters looms large. Byers (1998) and Ekblom and Åstrand (2000) argue strongly that biological drive for physical activity does exist. They suggest that the biological purpose of physical activity is more likely to be related to motor and neural development, and understanding how to enhance physical activity must go hand-in-hand with understanding the biological antecedents. The neural basis of physical activity is addressed in Rowland's (1998) eloquent review. He suggests the existence of a neural control mechanism or "activity-stat" which directs physical activity behaviour, and provides ample evidence to support the role of the central nervous system in this control process.

The idea that physical activity behaviour is controlled by a central biological process is given further support when investigations of neural damage and motor ability are considered. Stieh, Kramer, Harding, and Fischer (1999) provide evidence of abnormal motor function in children with cyanotic congenital heart disease, even after corrective surgery. The neurological basis for such impairment whilst not fully understood, is thought to be related to basal ganglia and ventral thalamus (Azzarelli, Caldemeyer, Phillips, & De Meyer, 1996; von Houten, Rothman, & Bejar, 1996). Motor development impairment in Stieh et al.'s (1999) study was also linked to poor cardiopulmonary function, and the authors conclude this was a result of reduced appropriate motor experiences limiting the differentiation of active behaviour. The exact role the central nervous system may play in the determination of physical activity in children is uncertain, however these data and data from hyperactive children (see Rowland, 1998) do suggest that a considerable influence exists. Whether the developmental changes in other aspects of function (e.g., ventilatory parameters), exert influence on physical activity patterns have received scant attention.

If we accept that a primary biological purpose of physical activity is to prepare and equip the young body to be motorically able, why then are children so inactive? Two possibilities can be suggested. First, physical activity levels have an upper limit in childhood. Rowland (1998) suggests that the "activity-stat" has a homeostatic optimum and above this optimal level, compensatory decreases in physical activity may actually occur. Data with children to support this explanation are few, but a recent study by Kriemler, Hebestreit, Mikami, et al. (1999) adds support to this possibility. They found high intensity activity caused a decrease in energy expenditure and time spent outdoors in obese boys the day following a regimented exercise bout. However, low to medium intensity exercise enhanced energy expenditure and time spent outdoors on the subsequent day in the same group of boys.

Second, our focus may be incorrect. Booth, Gordon, Carlson, and Hamilton (2000) argue that the physical inactivity levels, which characterize most of the objectively assessed childhood literature, are physiologically abnormal. Whilst the genome has remained largely the same, the phenotype has changed immeasurably as sedentary living has become the 'norm'. This is most clearly illustrated in Pima Indian communities in the USA and Mexico. Whilst genotypically identical, the sedentary lifestyle and poor dietary habits of those in the USA makes their obese phenotype a stark contrast to the slim one of the active Pima Indians in Mexico. When we study so-called 'normal' children, we are in effect studying an abnormally inactive group. Booth et al.'s (2000) argument concludes with the recommendation that if we want to understand the determinants of being a physically active child, we should study physically active children. They contend that if we work with our present 'normal' group, we should be careful to state that we are studying the effects of physical inactivity as opposed to physical activity. In essence the available data are not generally from 'normal' children. This second possibility is given some support by work looking at the relationship between physical activity and aerobic fitness in physically active adolescents (Mirwald, Bailey, Cameron, & Rasmussen, 1981). However, this relationship did not exist when the physically active boys were prepubertal, suggesting a maturational effect. Insufficient data exist which explore the influence of being a habitually physically active child upon markers of fitness or optimal growth and development. Booth's et al.'s (2000) proposition does however deserve further attention in the young.

Whilst it is accepted that physical activity has a primary biological purpose, when put into the context of the various extraneous factors that influence behaviour, it may come as no surprise to find an inactive population. There are many pressures on young people in Hong Kong:

environmental; an overemphasis on academic achievement at the expense of all-round development (Tsoi & Pryde, 1999); differential experiences mediated by a strongly engendered culture and a lack of interest by Hong Kong society in cultivating a want to be physically active. A thorough understanding of the theoretically relevant cultural and environmental variables underpinning physical activity behaviour is needed.

Despite a number of studies documenting levels of physical activity in Hong Kong children, we are still far from a complete understanding of what determines physical activity, or what effect physical activity has upon growth and development or health in the Chinese child. No systematic study of the biological control of physical activity has been attempted in children and only by integrating biological study with contextual and cultural study are answers going to emerge.

References

Armstrong, N., Kirby, B., McManus, A., & Welsman, J. (1995). Peak oxygen uptake in pre-pubescent children. *Annals of Human Biology, 22,* 427–441.

Armstrong, N., Welsman, J. R., & Kirby, B. J. (2000). Longitudinal changes in 11–13 year olds' physical activity. *Acta Paediatrica, 89,* 775–780.

Åstrand, P. O. (1952*). Experimental studies of physical working capacity in relation to sex and age.* Copenhagen: Muskgaard.

Azzarelli, B., Caldemeyer, K. S., Phillips, J. P., & De Meyer, W. E. (1996). Hypoxic-ischemic encephalopathy in areas of primary myelination: A neuroimaging and PET study. *Pediatric Neurology, 14,* 108–116.

Banerjee, B. & Saha, N. (1982). Energy cost of some common physical activities of Chinese schoolboys. *Annals of Nutrition and Metabolism, 26,* 360–366.

Barnett, A., Chan, L. Y. S., & Bruce, I. C. (1993). A preliminary study of the 20-m multistage shuttle run as a predictor of peak oxygen uptake in Hong Kong Chinese students. *Pediatric Exercise Science, 5,* 44–48.

Barnett, A., Bacon-Shone, J., Tam, K. H., Leung, M., Armstrong, N. (1995). Peak oxygen uptake of 12–18 year-old boys living in a densely populated urban environment. *Annals of Human Biology, 22,* 525–532.

Berman, N., Bailey, R., Barstow, T. J., & Cooper, D. M. (1998). Spectral and bout detection analysis of physical activity patterns in healthy, prepubertal boys and girls. *American Journal of Human Biology, 10,* 289–297.

Beunen, G., & Malina, R. M. (1988). Growth and physical performance relative to the timing of the adolescent spurt. *Exercise and Sport Science Reviews, 16,* 503–540.

Beunen, G., Ostyn, M., Simons, J., et al. (1997). Development and tracking in fitness components: Leuven longitudinal study on lifestyle, fitness and health. *International Journal of Sports Medicine, 18* (Suppl 3):s171–s178.

Booth, F. W, Gordon. S. E., Carlson, C. J., & Hamilton, M. T. (2000). Waging war on modern diseases: primary prevention through exercise biology. *Journal of Applied Physiology, 88,* 774–787.

Byers, J. A. (1998). The biology of human play. *Child Development, 69,* 599–600.

Chan, W. K., Chiu, A., Ko, G. T., et al. (1999). Ten-year cardiovascular risk in a Hong Kong population. *Journal of Cardiovascular Risk, 6,* 163–169.

Chan, W.S., & Hui, S. C. (2000). Evaluation of three physical activity questionnaires in predicting cardiovascular fitness of Chinese children. In *Proceedings of the International Conference of Physical Education* (pp. 493–497). Hong Kong: Hong Kong Institute of Education.

Cheng, C. H., McManus, A., & Macfarlane, D. (2002). Cardio-respiratory adjustment to training in 9-11 year old Chinese boys. Paper presented at the 7th Annual Conference of the European College of Sport Science, Athens, Greece.

Eisenmann, J. C., Malina, R. M. (2002). Secular trend in peak oxygen consumption among United States Youth in the 20th Century. *American Journal of Human Biology, 14,* 699–706.

Ekblom, B., & Astrand, P. O. (2000). Role of physical activity on health in children and adolescents. *Acta Paediatrica, 89,* 762–774.

Eston, R. G., Ingledew, D. K., Fu, F. H., & Rowlands, A. (1998). Comparison of health-related fitness measures in 7- to- 15- year olds in Hong Kong and North Wales. In K. M. Chan & L. J. Micheli (Eds.), *Sports and children* (pp. 119–130). Hong Kong: Williams and Wilkins Asia-Pacific.

Gilbey, H, & Gilbey, M. (1995). The physical activity of Singapore primary school children as estimated by heart rate monitoring. *Pediatric Exercise Science, 7,* 26–35.

Government of Hong Kong Home Affairs Bureau (2002). *Sports policy review.* Hong Kong: Author.

Haennel, R. G., & Lemire, F. (2002). Physical activity to prevent cardiovascular disease. How much is enough? *Canadian Family Physician, 48,* 65–71.

Hardman, A. E. (1999). Accumulation of physical activity for health gains: What is the evidence? *British Journal of Sports Medicine, 33,* 87–92.

Hatano, Y., Hua, Z. D., Jiang, L. D., Fu, F., Zhi, C. J., & Wei, S. D. (1997). Comparative study of physical fitness of the youth in Asia and their attitude toward sports. *Journal of Physical Education and Recreation (Hong Kong), 3,* 4–11.

Hu, G., Pekkarinen, H., Hanninen, O., Yu, Z., Gui, Z., & Tian, H. G. (2002). Commuting, leisure-time physical activity and cardiovascular risk factors in China. *Medicine and Science in Sports and Exercise, 34,* 234–238.

Ji, C. Y. (2001). Age at spermarche and comparison of growth and performance of pre- and post-spermarchael Chinese boys. *American Journal of Human Biology, 13,* 35–43.

Johns, D. P., & Ha, A. S. (1999). Home and recess physical activity of Hong Kong children. *Research Quarterly for Exercise and Sport, 70,* 319–323.

Kriemler, S., Hebestreit, H., Mikami, S., Bar-Or, T., Ayub, B. V., & Bar-Or, O. (1999). Impact of a single exercise bout on energy expenditure and spontaneous physical activity of obese boys. *Pediatric Research, 46,* 40–44.

Leung, S. S. F., Chan, Y. L., Lam, C. W. K, Peng, X. H., Woo, K. S., & Metreweli, C. (1998). Body fatness and serum lipids of 11-year-old Chinese children. *Acta Paediatrica, 87,* 363–367.

Lindner, K. J. (1998). Sport and physical activity participation of Hong Kong school children and youth. *Hong Kong Journal of Sports Medicine and Sport Science, 6,* 16–28.

Louie, L., Eston, R., Rowlands, A. V., Tong, K. K., Ingledew, D. K., & Fu, F. H. (1999). Validity of heart rate, pedometer and accelerometer for estimating the energy cost of activity in Hong Kong Chinese boys. *Pediatric Exercise Science, 11,* 229–239.

Macau Education and Youth Department (2000). *Physique and fitness of adolescents in Macau.* Report for the Macau Education and Youth Department. Macau: Government of the SAR of Macau.

Macfarlane, D. J. (1997). Some disturbing trends in the level of habitual physical activity in Hong Kong primary children: Preliminary findings. *Hong Kong Journal of Sports Medicine and Sports Science, 5,* 42–46.

Mackelvie, K. J., Mckay, H. A., Khan, K. M., & Crocker, P. R. E. (2001) Lifestyle risk factors for osteoporosis in Asian and Caucasian girls. *Medicine and Science in Sports and Exercise, 33,* 1818–1824.

Matsudo, V. K. R. (1996). Prediction of future athlete excellence. In O. Bar-

Or (Ed.), *The child and adolescent athlete* (pp. 92–112). Oxford, UK: Blackwell Science.

Matthews, C. E., Shu, X. O., Jin, F., Dai, Q., Herbert, J. R., Ruan, Z. X., Gao, Y. T., & Zheng, W. (2001). Lifetime physical activity and breast cancer risk in the Shanghai Breast Cancer Study. *British Journal of Cancer, 84,* 994–1001.

McKay, H. A., Petit, M. A., Khan, K. M., & Schutz, R. W. (2000). Lifestyle determinants of bone mineral: a comparison between prepubertal Asian-Canadian and Caucasian-Canadian boys and girls. *Calcified Tissue International, 66,* 320–324.

McManus, A., & Armstrong, N. (1996a). Inactivity of male and female children. In D. J. Macfarlane (Ed.), *Gender issues in sport and exercise. Proceedings of the 6th Conference organised by the University of Hong Kong Centre for Physical Education and Sport and the Physical Education and Sport Science Unit* (pp. 35–39). Hong Kong: The University of Hong Kong.

McManus, A., & Armstrong, N. (1996b). The peak oxygen uptake of Hong Kong Chinese children. *The Physiologist, 39,* A-24.

McManus, A., Hung, N., & Yung, T. C. (2002). Exercise testing in Chinese children with congenital heart defects. In *Proceedings of the 12th Commonwealth International Sport Conference* (p. 246). Manchester.

Mirwald , R. L., Bailey, D. A., Cameron, N., & Rasmussen, R. L. (1981). Longitudinal comparison of aerobic power in active and inactive boys aged 7.0 to 17.0 years. *Annals of Human Biology, 8,* 405–414.

National Institute of Health (1996). Consensus development panel on physical activity and cardiovascular health. *Journal of the American Medical Association, 276,* 241–246.

Ng, I. K. W. (1996). Physical activity patterns of Hong Kong adolescents. *Journal of Physical Education and Recreation (HK), 4,* 61–66.

Ohsawa, S., Ji, C. Y., & Kasai, N. (1997). Age at menarche and comparison of the growth and performance of pre-and post-menarcheal girls in China. *American Journal of Human Biology, 9,* 205–212.

Rowland, T. W. (1998). The biological basis of physical activity. *Medicine and Science in Sports and Exercise, 30,* 392–399.

Rowlands, A. V., Eston, R., Louie, L., Ingledew, D. K., Tong, K. K., & Fu, F. H. (2002). Physical activity levels of Hong Kong Chinese children: Relationship with body fat. *Pediatric Exercise Science, 14,* 286–296.

Sallis, J. F., & Patrick, K. (1994). Physical activity guidelines for adolescents: a consensus statement. *Pediatric Exercise Science, 6,* 890–895.

Schmidt, G. J., Stensel, D. J., & Walkuski, J. J. (1997). Blood pressure, lipids, lipoproteins, body fat and physical activity of Singapore children. *Journal of Paediatrics and Child Health, 33,* 484–490.

Stieh, J., Kramer, H. H., Harding, P., & Fischer, G. (1999). Gross and fine motor development is impaired in children with cyanotic congenital heart disease. *Neuropediatrics, 30,* 77–82.

Tong, T. K., Fu, F. H., & Chow, B. C. (2002). Reliability of a 5-min running field test and its accuracy in VO$_2$max evaluation. *Journal of Sports Medicine and Physical Fitness, 41,* 318–323.

Tsoi, M. M., Pryde, N. A. (1999). Hong Kong's children: overview and conclusion. In N. A. Pryde & M. M. Tsoi (Eds.), *Hong Kong's children: Our past, their future* (pp. 13–20). Hong Kong: Centre of Asian Studies Occasional Papers and Monographs No. 137, University of Hong Kong.

Von Houten, J. P., Rothman, A., & Bejar, R. (1996). High incidence of cranial ultrasound abnormalities in full term infants with congenital heart disease. *American Journal of Perinatology, 13,* 47–53.

Wong, T. K. (1997). Aspects of habitual physical activity in Hong Kong primary school children. Unpublished M.Phil. Thesis, The University of Hong Kong.

Wong, T. W., Yu, T. S., Wang, X. R., & Robinson, P. (2001). Predicted maximal oxygen uptake in normal Hong Kong Chinese schoolchildren and those with respiratory disease. *Pediatric Pulmonology, 31,* 126–132.

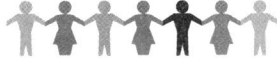

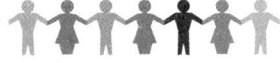

CHAPTER 6

Involvement of Hong Kong Youth in Physical Activity and Sport: Extent, Motives and Participation Factors

Cindy Sit Hui Ping, Ken Chow Chi Kin, and Koenraad J. Lindner

Introduction

As the title of this book intimates, there is a link between children's wellbeing and the amount of physical activity they engage in. Inactive children's wellness is threatened in a number of ways. They are more likely to become overweight or obese with all the associated health risks discussed in other chapters in this volume (Sung & Nelson, Chapter 7; Thomas, Chan, Cockram, & Tomlinson, Chapter 8). They are also at risk of becoming sedentary, unfit, motorically awkward grown-ups, since physical inactivity tends to track into adulthood (e.g., Yang, Telama, & Laakso, 1996): Lazy kids are likely to be lazy adults. They also miss out on the potentials for enjoyment, pride and learning that physical activities and sports provide. One can never appreciate the joy and satisfaction of achieving something through hard physical effort if one never engages in such effort. In short, inactive children are unnaturally pitiable as well as a source for serious future health concerns.

It is against this background that research in children's physical activity levels takes on its great importance. We need to know the extent of the current problem (Hong Kong children's sedentary lifestyle) and to anticipate the coming consequences (the future state of the health of the population). We also need this information to monitor further developments: Is the problem getting worse, or, are interventions successful? In this chapter we examine and summarize findings from our research on children's and youth's physical activity participation over the past decade. We will present the self-reported extent of involvement in sport and exercise derived from a number of surveys since 1993 to demonstrate that our data are in line with results from other studies with different methods (e.g., Macfarlane, 1997; McManus & Armstrong, 1996), namely that Hong Kong children are insufficiently active and that this seems to be getting worse over time. We will search for possible causes for this by analyzing motives for participation and non participation in physical activity among Hong Kong youth, and by examining factors that relate to participation and to intentions for future participation.

Self-reported Extents of Participation in Physical Activities

Yearly surveys conducted by the former Physical Education and Sports Science Unit (now the Institute of Human Performance) of the University of Hong Kong over the past decade have generated a large volume of data pertaining to physical activity participation. In each survey we asked respondents to estimate their own frequency of engaging in sport or exercise in the past year, discounting the school's physical education classes. While frequency by itself is a rather crude measure of physical activity participation, it is probably reliable enough to determine who is active and who is not. We have used other measures as well, such as indices based on frequency, duration and number of months per year (Lindner, 1998), but the outcome and conclusions have always been consistently similar. The missing of the exercise intensity ingredient in the indices makes our measurement of physical activity unsuitable for drawing of medical and physiological conclusions, but for the purpose of estimating what percentage of the population is sedentary or active, the frequency variable is assumed to be adequate.

In Tables 1 and 2 we have simplified the data by reducing frequency of participation to three categories, i.e., those who never or seldom

Table 1. Percentages of elementary and secondary school respondents in participation frequency categories by gender in three different samples

Participation frequency	BOYS				GIRLS			
	1996 Disabled Up Prim/Sec N = 143	1996 Upper Primary N = 763	1996 Secondary N = 1,518	1999 Secondary N = 1,799	1996 Disabled Up Prim/Sec N = 92	1996 Upper Primary N = 855	1996 Secondary N = 2,115	1999 Secondary N = 1,198
Never/Seldom	45	26	27	33	60	34	53	70
Regularly	18	12	12	28	15	15	19	18
(Very) Often	36	62	61	39	24	51	28	12

Table 2. Percentages of university entrants in participation frequency categories by gender in four different samples

Participation frequency	MALES				FEMALES			
	1993 HKU N = 1,338	1996 HKU N = 1,435	1999 HKU N = 713	2000 HKU N = 690	1993 HKU N = 1,442	1996 HKU N = 1,679	1999 HKU N = 964	2000 HKU N = 889
Never/Seldom	54	37	36	34	62	61	65	64
Regularly	32	47	37	42	31	31	24	25
(Very) Often	14	16	27	24	7	8	12	11

engage in physical activity (a few times per month or less), those who participate on a regular basis (2 to 3 times per week), and those who are often involved (more than 3 times per week).

The samples in Table 1 are from two large surveys of school children (Lindner, 1997, 2001) conducted with funding from the Hong Kong Sports Development Board and a grant from the Research Grant Commission, and a smaller study of physical activity participation by school children with disabilities (Sit, 1998; Sit & Lindner, 1998, 2000; Sit, Lindner, & Sherrill, 2002). The data for the upper primary children appear reasonably acceptable with two-thirds of the boys and one-half of the girls in the 'often' category. However, it is worrisome that a quarter of the primary boys and one-third of the girls were not or rarely physically active outside the PE classes. The results for the secondary school respondents were even more alarming, particularly for the girls. For both genders there was a large decline in the percentages in the '(very) often' group from 1996 to 1999, while the inactive proportion of girls rose from 53 to 70%. It was reported previously (Lindner, 1998) that the activity level of boys does not change appreciably between the ages of 8 and 18 years, whereas the girls' participation drops sharply. The implication here is that compared to the 1996 cohort, the 1999 cohort as a whole is significantly less active. Future study must establish whether this negative trend is continuing. The results for the disabled children will be discussed in a later section.

The samples in Table 2 are all from annual surveys of students entering university and therefore reporting on their frequency of participation in the year before being admitted to HKU. Most of these are therefore indicating their activity level in the last year of high school. One would expect these samples to be different from the general school population, since these were among the elite students. Previous studies (Lindner, 1999, 2002) have shown that the better academic students tend to be also the ones that are more physically active. However, it can be argued that in their year of examinations they would have less opportunity to engage in sport and exercise. The participation levels of the females were consistent over the four surveys presented here in that about two-thirds of them do not or rarely participate in physical activity. For the males this is slightly over one-third, and there is a small improvement detectable over the seven years the surveys covered. Significant differences in participation extents have been reported between genders, among age levels, and among regions of Hong Kong (Lindner, 1998), and among schools with different band ratings (Lindner, 2001).

The above data are indicative of the low levels of physical activity in Hong Kong children and youth. About one-third of all upper elementary school children and secondary school males are sedentary, while between 60 and 70% of secondary school female students are inactive. We are also concerned that these data probably represent under-estimations. First, it is more likely that they are subject to over-reporting (i.e., the respondents indicating a higher category of activity frequency than warranted) than to under-reporting. Second, since only frequency is considered and not duration and intensity, there is no way to allay the probability that much of the reported activity falls below levels of intensity that constitute a health benefit.

Motives for Participation in Physical Activity

It is important for a number of reasons to establish why children and youth engage in sport and physical activities. Lindner (1995) argued that too often sport managers, educators and scientists theorized why kids participate and what they should be getting out of sport involvement, without paying much attention to the subjective experiences of kids themselves. Examining motives for participation, non-participation and withdrawal demonstrates the possible reasons why children remain, avoid or drop out of sport. Theories such as competence motivation (Harter, 1978, 1981) and achievement goal orientation (Nicholls, 1984) have not been helpful in promoting mass participation. The error was to generalize findings from studies on competitive sport participants to all physical activity participants. The assumption that children are physically active because they want to achieve something actually applies only to the relatively few (especially in Hong Kong) serious competitive sport participants. The rest have other reasons for engaging in sport and exercise, such as fun derived from playing together with friends, wanting to be fitter, or to meet expectations set by parents or others. For these participants serious training to improve skills and efforts to win in competition are not attractive objectives, and they will avoid entering such contexts, or quickly leave them.

To demonstrate that sport excellence and skill development are not primary motives for many children, we examined the ratings respondents assigned to various motives in relation to their perceived physical ability (PPA). In our surveys we ask respondents to rate their own ability in sport and physical activity on a Likert scale. We then determined the relative importance of participation motives for PPA groups. The results are presented in Table 3 for school samples and in Table 4 for university entrants (the 'average' PPA groups are omitted). In the 1996 school sample (Lindner & Sit, 1999) only three choices were presented (Above average, AA; Average; and Below average, BA). The BA groups were clearly more motivated by fun with friends than by being or wanting to become good at the activity. Interestingly, when more ability groupings were available in the 1999 survey, 'becoming good' had high rankings in both the FAA and the FBA groups, whereas the other groups aimed at 'fitness' and 'fun', respectively.

Similarly, skill and sport excellence ranked higher for the higher ability groups in the 1993 HKU sample (Lindner & Speak, 1995), but the main objective for the university entrants were health and enjoyment (Table 4). In the 1999 HKU sample fitness and fun were again the strongest reasons for all ability groups with 'becoming good' slightly more important for the FAA group. ANOVA analyses showed that differences among PPA groups were large and highly significant for the 'become good', 'skill', and 'sport excellence' reasons, but much smaller for the other motives (Lindner & Sit, 1999; Lindner & Speak, 1995).

It is clear from the above results that, for some of the physical activity participants, achievements in skill and sport prowess are principal motives for involvement. Many organized sport contests including those provided by the schools, fail to recognize that youngsters express fun, fitness and friends as the primary reasons for their involvement and as a consequence do not consider these motivations in their programmes. This could well be one of the major factors contributing to the low participation in and high attrition from physical activities observed in Hong Kong.

Table 3. Ranks of participation motives in perceived physical ability groups for two school samples

1996 School Sample				1999 School sample				
Motive	FBA	BA	AA	FAA	Motive	FBA	BA	AA	FAA
Fit/Healthy		3	3		Fit/Healthy	1	1	1	2*
Fun/Enjoy		1	2		Fun/Enjoy	3	2	2	2*
Become good		4	1		Become good	2	3	3	1
Good at it		6	4		Cooperation	4	4	4*	5
Friends		2	5		Help others	6	5	4*	4
Praise		7	6		Appreciation	5	6	6	6
Told to		5	7		Expected	8	7	7	8
					Rebellious	7	8	8	7

FBA = Far below average, BA = Below average, AA = Above average, FAA = Far above average
* tied ratings

Table 4. Ranks of participation motives in perceived physical ability groups for two HKU samples

1993 HKU Sample					1999 HKU sample				
Motive	FBA	BA	AA	FAA	Motive	FBA	BA	AA	FAA
Health	1	1	2	3	Fit/Healthy	1	1	1	2
Leisure/Enjoy	2	2	1	1	Fun/Enjoy	2	2	2	1
Skill	3	4	3	2	Become good	4	4	4	3
Sport Excel	7	7	5	4	Cooperation	3	3	3	4
Friends	4	3	4	5	Help others	7	6	5	5
Character	5	5	6	7	Appreciation	8	5	6	6
Image	6	6	7	6	Expected	6	8	7	7
					Rebellious	5	7	8	8

FBA = Far below average, BA = Below average, AA = Above average, FAA = Far above average

Participation by Hong Kong Children and Youth with Disabilities

Research on sport participation has been identified as one of the key topics in disability sport (DePauw, 1986; Doll-Tepper, 1998). Past Western literature indicates that children with disabilities are in general sedentary and that demographic variables such as gender, age, or disability influence their participation in sport and physical activity (Longmuir & Bar-Or, 1994, 2000). Little research has however been done to examine this area in children with disabilities in a local context. This line of research is particularly important if practitioners working with children with disabilities wish to encourage children's sport participation, for the purpose of developing healthier and more active lifestyles and maximizing opportunities for empowerment (Hutzler & Sherrill, 1999).

Sit and Lindner (1998) conducted a comparative study to determine the sport participation patterns and motives between children with and without disabilities. Participants comprised children without disabilities ($N = 4690$), data generated in the studies reported by Lindner (1998) and Lindner and Sit (1999); and children with disabilities ($N = 237$) attending special schools (Sit, 1998). Five types of disabilities were included: physical disability, visual impairment, hearing impairment, mild mental disability, and maladjustment. Results indicated that there were similarities in sport participation frequency and patterns between these two groups. The data presented in Table 1 indicate slightly lower participation frequency for the boys, but comparable figures for the girls. There was no evidence to support the stereotyped notion that children with disabilities are substantially less active due to their disabilities. This group also demonstrated a higher number of sport club membership and a lower sport dropout rate, as well as a greater strengths of sport participation motives, when compared to the children without disabilities.

In view of the importance motivation theories attached to the perception of one's physical ability for sport participation, Sit and Lindner (2000) examined the sport participation motivation of both children with and without disabilities who differed in their levels of perceived physical ability (PPA). It was found that children with disabilities of higher PPA level were more motivated by competence-related and social motives for sport participation than children without disabilities of same PPA level. Children with disabilities of lower PPA level, however, perceived participation motives of achievement and competence as less important, and 'injury' as a more important withdrawal motive, when compared to their able-bodied counterparts. This study suggests that lower PPA level may indicate that a fragile self-concept is a more powerful influencing factor and that PPA, instead of disability, could be a stronger predictor of participation motivation of children with disabilities. It also yielded the same conclusion as for the able-bodies sample, i.e., that skill achievement was more important to children with disabilities with high PPA than those with low PPA.

A comprehensive study conducted by Sit et al. (2002) further investigated the influence of demographic variables, namely, gender, two school levels, and five disability types on sport participation patterns and motivation in children with disabilities. Results relating to participation frequency and extent demonstrated that girls were less active than boys and that children with physical disability, visual impairment, and mental disability were less active than children with hearing impairment and maladjustment.

Demographic variables such as gender, school level, and disability type were also significant in affecting children's sport motives in this study. The praise motive was important for girls. Older children on the other hand perceived fitness as a significant sport motive, "other achievements" as non participation motive, and "doing other fun things" as withdrawal motive. Children with mental disability were driven by the achievement- or competence-related sport and withdrawal motives, children with visual impairment by the achievement sport motive, children with hearing impairment by both achievement and social sport motives, and children with physical disability by the skill-related and injury nonparticipation and withdrawal motives.

This study generally concluded that disability type is considered to be the most significant variable that influences both sport participation patterns and motivation in children with disabilities. How children perceive the existing barriers to and opportunities for sport participation as well as their real or perceived limitations would vary by different types of disabilities. Special emphasis should therefore be placed on disability type difference when we determine the sporting needs or motives in children with disabilities.

Factors Affecting Intended and Actual Physical Activity Participation

In addition to assessing the extent of and the reasons for participation in sport and exercise, it is important to identify the factors that contribute to children's engagement in physical activity. In recent studies Chow and Lindner (2000) and Chow (2002) examined the interrelationships among psychological, social and situational factors in children's physical activity participatory behaviour in the framework of Ajzen's Theory of Planned Behavior (Ajzen, 1985, 1987). Specifically, the roles of self factors (such as attitude towards physical activity, perceived physical competence and past participatory behaviour), parental factors (such as encouragement, enjoyment and role-modeling), and situational factors (perceived resources and familial support) in the prediction of intended and actual physical activity participation were estimated through complex modeling techniques (structural equation modeling). Intended activity participation was quantified through questionnaire items representing frequency, duration and vigor of intention of physical activity in the next two weeks. Actual participation was calculated from responses to the same items in a follow-up questionnaire. Measures of attitude, parental factors and perceived control were made via a modified existing instrument (Children's Attraction to Physical Activity, CAPA; Brustad, 1993, 1996). The sample comprised 1,920 primary and secondary school students in Hong Kong and 1,043 of their parents or guardians who responded to a separate parental questionnaire inquiring about their attitude toward physical activity, their own physical competence, what they believed the physical competence of their child was, their own extent of physical activity participation, and the extent to which they encouraged participation by their child. Factor analyses of these responses yielded eight factors from the children's 50 questionnaire items and nine from the parental 40 items.

Findings

The main results from the structural equation modeling procedures are summarized in Table 5. The child's attitude and perceived physical competence were the main predictors of intention for physical activity participation, but competence and past participatory behavior were found to have direct effects on actual participation in the whole sample (attitude only for the 10–11 years old). The factor 'subjective norm' (comprising parental encouragement, enjoyment and role-modeling) was a significant positive contributor to actual participation in 12–15 year old girls, but had a slightly negative influence in the whole sample. Interestingly, the subjective norm was a significant negative force on intention for children with parents who had a low attitude towards physical activity participation, but a significant positive effect on actual participation for those whose parents had a positive attitude. In addition, youngsters' self-perceived physical competence was associated with how they thought their parents perceived their child's competence, and the parents' perception of their own (parents') competence was highly correlated with how they perceived their child's competence. This means that the higher the child's self-perception of competence is, the higher they thought their parents would rate them, and the more competent the parent felt, the more competent they thought their children were.

The situational factor, representing opportunities for engaging in physical activity had a stronger effect on girls' intention for

Table 5. Factors significantly associated with intention to participate and actual participation in a sample of school children and youth (Chow, 2002)

	Intention for Participation	Actual Participation
Self Factors	+ Attitude toward PA* (all) + Physical Competence (all)	+ Physical Competence (all) + Past PA Behavior (all) + Attitude (10–11y)
Parental Factors	– Selective Norm (Low-attitude parents)	+ Subjective Norm (girls 12–15y) + Subjective Norm (high-attitude parents)
Situational Factors	+ Perceived External Control (girls > boys)	+ Availability/Access (high perceived external control)

participation than their self-perceived competence did, whereas boys were more affected by physical competence than by perceived external resources in their attention to be physically active. Availability and access to resources had a significant direct effect on actual physical activity participation, particularly for those who rated the external control high.

When the model was tested for boys and girls separately, and for different age levels, it became evident that self, parental and situational factors interact differently on intention for physical activity participation and actual participation for boys and girls and for all age groups. For example, there was an increase with age in the effect of attitude on intention, whereas the effect of perceived competence decreased. So attitude became more important than feelings of competence with increasing age, but competence remained more influential for boys than for girls.

When asked in the follow-up instrument to rank reasons for more or less physical activity than they had predicted two weeks before in the initial questionnaire, the main reasons the respondents provided were as listed in Table 6. Availability of someone to play with and study pressures featured among the most important ones.

Table 6. The five highest ranked reasons for less than and more than intended physical activity participation (Chow 2002)

Rank	Less than intended	More than intended
1	Needed time for studying	I had a peer companion
2	Lack of peer companion	My skill improved
3	Have other interests or hobbies	Better time arrangement
4	Weather constraints	Want to be healthier
5	Interest in physical activity declined	Enhanced confidence

Implications

Attitude towards physical activity appears to play an important role in intention for and actual participation in physical activity, including the attitude of the parents. Poor attitude of parents had a negative effect on the child's intention to participate, whereas a good attitude positively influenced actual participation. Together with perceived competence (particularly for the boys), past participation behavior and own and parental attitudes appear to form a strong effect on participation. Parents' and student's perceptions of physical competence were also related, as were parents' and students' attitudes toward physical activity. It is reasonable to conclude that the physically active child in this study tended to have (a) a habit of being physically active, (b) a positive attitude toward physical activity, (c) parents who had a positive attitude, (d) a positive perception of his or her own physical abilities, and (e) parents who had a positive perception of their own and their child's physical competence. This implies an acceptance of physical activity as an important aspect of life by the children and their families. Children who have good attitude and are physically active can be expected to become parents with the same characteristics, thus starting or perpetuating a culture of an active lifestyle. Children not so advantaged would have to achieve a desirable lifestyle without or even against the parental influences, and would need help to strengthen their competence feelings and attitudes, a role eminently suited to appropriate programmes of school physical education.

The Role of Perceived Competence in Physical Activity Participation

Chow's (2002) study showed that perceived physical competence was strongly associated in a positive sense with physical activity participatory behaviour: good competence feelings predicted good intention for and good actual participation. From Sit's and Lindner's results it was concluded, however, that physical competence was not a major reason for participation for many of the respondents. These seemingly contradictory findings are easily reconcilable when one realizes that physical competence was a measured (perceived) quality of the respondents in Chow's study, but a desired outcome in the Sit and Lindner studies: those respondents who rated themselves high in physical abilities rated skill and sport excellence motives higher than those with low perceived ability, who preferred other outcomes, such as fitness or social benefits. For future developments in physical education curricula it is important to recognize that perceived physical competence is not synonymous with high skill level or sports excellence. While skilled athletes generally have high feelings of physical competence, they are not the only ones. Physical competence needs to be seen as much broader concept, encompassing general capabilities for regulating physical activity for health and fitness. In particular, youngsters need to be acquainted with the rationale for selecting activities that develop motor control, the knowledge required for participating at a functional level, and the understanding that provides for feeling at ease in and deriving enjoyment from physical activity contexts. Many students will never be or feel competent in sport skills, but all can attain a perception of physical competence in this broader sense. School physical education in particular must adapt its curriculum to this broader interpretation of 'physical competence'.

References

Ajzen, I. (1985). From intentions to actions: A theory of planned behavior. In J. Kuhl & J. Beckmann (Eds.), *Action-control: From cognition to behavior* (pp. 11–39). Heidelberg: Springer.

Ajzen, I. (1987). Attitudes, traits, and action: Dispositional prediction of behavior in personality and social psychology. In L. Berkowitz (Ed.), *Advances in experimental social psychology* (Vol. 20, pp. 1–63). New York: Academic Press.

Brustad, R. J. (1993). Who will go out and play? Parental and psychological influences on children's attraction to physical activity. *Pediatric Exercise Science, 5,* 210–223.

Brustad, R. J. (1996). Attraction to physical activity in urban school children: Parental socialization and gender influences. *Research Quarterly for Exercise and Sport, 67,* 316–323.

Chow, C. K. K. (2002). *Perceived self, parental and situational factors in physical activity participatory behavior of Hong Kong children and youth: A test of Ajzen's Theory of Planned Behavior.* Ph.D. dissertation, The University of Hong Kong.

Chow, C. K. K., & Lindner, K. J. (2000). Testing Ajzen's Theory of Planned Behavior on the physical activity participatory behavior of Hong Kong children and youth: A pilot study. In M. K. Chin, L. D. Hensley, & Y. K. Liu (Eds.), *Innovation and application of physical education and sports science in the new millennium — An Asia-Pacific perspective* (pp. 373–386). Hong Kong: The Hong Kong Institute of Education.

DePauw, K. (1986). Research on sport for athletes with disabilities. *Adapted Physical Activity Quarterly, 3*, 292–299.

Doll-Tepper, G. (1998). *International perspectives on research in adapted physical activity.* Paper presented at the AIESEP World Congress, Garden City, New York, July 13–17.

Harter, S. (1978). Effectance motivation reconsidered. *Human Development, 21*, 34–64.

Harter, S. (1981). A model of intrinsic mastery motivation in children: Individual differences and developmental change. In W. A. Collins (Ed.), *Minnesota symposium on child psychology, Vol. 14* (pp. 215–255). Hillsdale, NJ: Erlbaum.

Hutzler, Y., & Sherrill, C. (1999). Disability, physical activity, psychological well-being and empowerment: A life-span perspective. In R. Lidor & M. Bar-Eli (Eds.), *Sport psychology: Linking theory and practice* (pp. 281–300). Morgantown, WV: Fitness Information Technology.

Lindner, K. J. (1995). Motivational factors in the promotion of sport participation. *Hong Kong Journal of Sports Medicine and Sports Science, 6*, 16–27.

Lindner, K. J. (1997). *Sport participation by Hong Kong children and youth: Rates and reasons.* Report to the Hong Kong Sports Development Board. Hong Kong: The University of Hong Kong.

Lindner, K. J. (1998). Sport participation by Hong Kong children and youth: Part I: Extent and nature of participation. *The Hong Kong Journal of Sports Medicine and Sports Science, 6*, 16–27.

Lindner, K. J. (1999). Sport participation and perceived academic performance of school children and youth. *Pediatric Exercise Science, 10*, 129–143.

Lindner, K. J. (2001). Banding effects in physical activity participation extent and reasons therefor of Hong Kong secondary school pupils. *Hong Kong Journal of Sports Medicine and Sports Science, 12*, 21–33.

Lindner, K. J. (2002). The activity participation — academic performance relationship revisited: Perceived and actual performance, and the effect of banding (academic tracking). *Pediatric Exercise Science, 14*, 155–169.

Lindner, K. J., & Sit, C. H. P. (1999). Sport and activity participation of Hong Kong school children and youth: Part II: Reasons for participation, nonparticipation and withdrawal. *The Hong Kong Journal of Sports Medicine and Sports Science, 8,* 23–36.

Lindner, K. J., & Speak, M. A. (1995). Self-estimates of ability and fitness levels, and reasons for (non)participation by university entrants. In R. van Fraechem-Raway & Y. van den Auweele (Eds.), *Proceedings of the IXth European Congress on Sport Psychology, Part III* (pp. 1260–1267). Brussels: Universite Libre de Bruxelles.

Longmuir, P. E., & Bar-Or, O. (1994). Physical activity of children and adolescents with a disability: methodology and effects of age and gender. *Pediatric Exercise Science, 6,* 168–177.

Longmuir, P. E., & Bar-Or, O. (2000). Factors influencing the physical activity levels of youths with physical and sensory disabilities. *Adapted Physical Activity Quarterly, 17,* 40–53.

Macfarlane, D. J. (1997). Some disturbing trends in the level of habitual physical activity in Hong Kong primary school children: Preliminary findings. *Hong Kong Journal of Sports Medicine and Sports Science, 5,* 42–46.

McManus, A. M., & Armstrong, N. (1996). Physical activity patterns of Hong Kong primary school children. *Pediatric Exercise Science, 8,* 177–178.

Nicholls, J. G. (1984). Achievement motivation: Conceptions of ability, subjective experience, task choice, and performance. *Psychological Review, 91,* 328–346.

Sit, C. H. P. (1998). *Participation motivation in sport: A comparative study of able-bodied and disabled school-aged children in Hong Kong.* M. Phil. thesis, The University of Hong Kong.

Sit, C. H. P., & Lindner, K. J. (1998). *Sport participation motivation of able-bodied and disabled children in Hong Kong.* Paper presented at the AIESEP World Congress, Garden City, New York, July 13–17.

Sit, C. H. P., & Lindner, K. J. (2000). Perceived physical ability and sport participation of Hong Kong children with disabilities. *The Hong Kong Journal of Sports Medicine and Sports Science, 10,* 8–19.

Sit, C. H. P., Lindner, K. J., & Sherrill, C. (2002). Sport participation of Hong Kong Chinese children with disabilities in special schools. *Adapted Physical Activity Quarterly, 19,* 453–471.

Yang, X., Telama, R., & Laakso, L. (1996). Parents' physical activity, socioeconomic status and education as predictors of physical activity and sport among children and youths: A 12-year follow-up study. *International Review for the Sociology of Sport, 31,* 273–289.

PART III

Health Consequences of Lack of Physical Activity

The two chapters in Part III examine the increasingly more worrying trend of people in developed countries growing bigger and heavier. Overweight and obesity are now approaching prevalence figures in the Western world that have been labeled as 'pandemic'. Particularly the increase in overweight and obesity in children and youth is of great concern in view of their future health consequences and the enormous burden of health care costs on society.

Rita Sung and Tony Nelson describe the extent of the problem in Hong Kong in Chapter 7, and cite evidence for one of the suspected causes, namely the lack of physical activity. They then explain what health risks are associated with childhood obesity, including cardiovascular complications, Type-2 diabetes, sleep disorders, fatty liver and psychological effects.

In Chapter 8, Neil Thomas, Norman Chan, Clive Cockram and Brian Tomlinson present arguments for more stringent obesity criteria for Hong Kong Chinese than the WHO recommendations for European Caucasians. They present evidence for the implications of childhood obesity for adult health, and explain some of the mechanisms of obesity's impact on health, such as for central adiposity accumulation (how and why fat accumulates subcutaneously and among the viscera), insulin resistance and Type-2 diabetes (how obesity is linked to inadequate production of insulin and consequential abnormal blood sugar levels leading to a variety of health problems), hypertension (how obesity may be associated with high blood pressure), and dyslipidaemia (possible connections between obesity and fatty substances in the blood such as lipoproteins and cholesterol).

Both chapters have been included in order to provide a clinical perspective to support the concern over the prevalence of obesity among Hong Kong children and to indicate that physical activity is a major factor in the cause of, but also in the remedy for overweight and obesity.

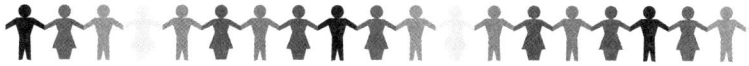

CHAPTER 7

Childhood Obesity: Possible Links to Inactivity and Health Risks

Rita Sung and Tony Nelson

What is the Contribution of Inactivity to Childhood Obesity?

The dramatic global increase in the prevalence of obesity is reaching epidemic proportions, in both developed and developing countries. The epidemic is affecting children as well as adults, with major health and economic implications (World Health Organization, 1998) Childhood and adolescent obesity is also a significant problem in Hong Kong where rates of obesity are increasing. A survey of 25,000 Hong Kong children in 1993 (Leung 1996) showed that 13.4% of boys and 10.5% of girls aged 6-18 years were obese (defined as >120% median weight-for-height using local reference ranges). Using the same definition, the Student Health Service of the Hong Kong Department of Health (personal communication) reported for 2000/2001 that 14.1% of all school children (6–18 years) were obese (primary school children: 17% males and 12% females; secondary school children: 12% males and 10% females). These data also showed that the overall rate of obesity had increased by 2% from a rate of 12.1% in 1997/1998 (Tong, personal communication).

While the causes for this surge are not entirely clear, a sedentary lifestyle is considered to be a major culprit. Western literature has shown that obese children are more sedentary than their non-obese counterparts in general. (Bar-Or, Foreyt, Bouchard, et al., 1998) Other studies have also shown that lifestyle factors such as television watching (Hernandez, Gortmaker, Colditz, et al., 1999) and inactivity (Fogelholm, Nuutinen, Pasanen, Myohanen, & Saatela, 1999; Obarzanek, Schreiber, Crawford, et al., 1994) are associated with childhood obesity development.

There are some data on habitual physical activity in Hong Kong children that have indicated that Hong Kong children are in general physically less active than their counterparts in the West (Fu & Hao, 2002; MacFarlane, 1997). A study of a stratified random sample of Hong Kong primary school children (primary class 3 to primary class 6, aged 8–12 years) measured activity over one normal school day using a 10- hour recording of heart rate (Polar Electro PE 4000) and accelerometry (Tritrac, Hemokinetics R3D). The results showed that only 24% of these children demonstrated a single-10 minute period where the heart rate was continuously above 139 beats/min (considered to reflect moderate physical activity) and only 4% demonstrated a similar period with heart rate continuously over 159 beats/min (considered to reflect vigorous physical activity). The corresponding figures for children who achieved a 20-minute period of continuous moderate and vigorous activities were 4% and 2% only. On average, Hong Kong children spent only 3.7% (27 minutes) of daytime with heart rate >139 beats/min. These proportions were the lowest among the available data from the United Kingdom (5.2%), USA (36 min), Singapore (38 min) (Macfarlane, 1997). More about this study in Chapter 8 of this book.

Another recent study using an activity diary and ambulatory heart rate monitoring method compared the time and energy expenditure in non-obese and obese children. The obese and non-obese children had similar basal metabolic rates when these were adjusted for fat-free mass and fat mass. The obese children spent 51% more time in sedentary activities. In addition they slept 12% less and spent 30% less time in physical activity. The mean ratio of physically active-to-sedentary waking time was 0.6 (± 0.4) in the obese compared to 1.9 (±2.2) (p = 0.021) in the non-obese children (Yu, Sung, So, et al., 2002).

A case-control study of 343 Hong Kong children aged 6–7 years old, used three body mass index (BMI) groups to identify possible risk factors for overweight (Hui, Nelson, Yu, Li, & Fok, 2003). The overweight group were children with a BMI $\geq 92^{nd}$ percentile, the normal middle-weight group had BMIs within the 45th–55th percentiles and a normal low-weight group had BMIs $\leq 8^{th}$ percentile. Subjects and their parents/caregivers were interviewed at home and data on lifestyle habits, dietary habits, family structure and demographic background were collected by questionnaire. A 3-day dietary record was administered to the parents/caregivers to assess dietary intake of the children. The results showed that there was no significant difference in the time spent on exercising, watching television or studying. However, sleeping duration (h/d) was negatively correlated with the child's weight. Heavier subjects tended to sleep less and a dose response effect between sleeping duration and overweight was shown with adjusted odds ratios (95% Confidence Intervals) of 0.54 (0.30–0.97) and 0.31(0.11–0.87 CF95%) for 9–11h/d and ≥ 11h/d, respectively. It has been suggested that this relationship may be the result of a hormonal mechanism, such as reduction of growth hormone secretion and increase in serum cortisol concentration. However at this stage it is not possible to determine whether overweight causes the lack of sleep, whether short sleeping duration results in weight gain, or whether the association is due to other confounding factors. No relationship was found between stated activity level and overweight but the study did support the results of other investigators that have shown that Hong Kong children are very inactive. Seventy-six percent of the subjects did not exercise during schooldays and 24% did not have regular exercise on both schooldays and holidays (weekends). The average time spent on watching television (2.8 ± 1.5 h/d) and studying (2.4 ± 1.1 h/d) were far more than that for exercise (0.4 ± 0.5 h/d). Thus although this study did not show a link between inactivity and overweight in these 6–7 year old children, it did confirm the general inactive behaviour in Hong Kong young children.

These studies show that Hong Kong children are generally physically inactive (both for overweight and normal weight) children and that there is some but not consistent evidence that this inactivity is related to overweight development. Two studies have also identified short sleep duration as a risk factor for overweight development although the association of sleep duration, physical activity and overweight is not well understood.

The Health Risks of Childhood Obesity

The adverse health effects of obesity on adult health and life expectancy is well recognised (World Health Organization, 1998). However it is increasingly being recognised that many of the health complications seen in adults are also being seen in children. The main complications of childhood obesity are cardiovascular and metabolic, obstructive sleep apnoea syndrome, steatohepatitis or fatty liver, orthopaedic problems and psychological effects.

Cardiovascular risk factors include what is termed the metabolic syndrome (high levels of insulin associated with obesity and increased risk of cardiovascular mortality) and direct effects on the body's vascular system. Local studies have shown that clustering of cardio-vascular risk factors is common in obese preadolescent children. A cross sectional study (Sung et al., 2003) of 271 obese and non-obese children showed that more than 77% of obese children and 20% of non-obese children had hyperinsulinemia. This high level of insulin is termed insulin resistance and it is a strong predictor of the future development of Type 2 diabetes and coronary heart disease. These results showing a the high prevalence of insulin resistance in these preadolescent children was of particular concern and is likely to have important public health implications in the future.

New measuring techniques with ultrasound are able to assess the responsiveness of arterial blood vessels. Poor response or what is termed arterial endothelial dysfunction has been demonstrated in obese Hong Kong children. Woo and colleagues studied 8 to 12 year-old overweight and obese children and found that they had impaired arterial endothelial function and increased thickness of the linings of the main carotid arteries in the neck (Woo, Chook, Yu, et al, 2001).

Sleep apnoea has long been recognised as a complication of severe obesity in children, the so-called Pickwickian Syndrome. However, lesser degrees of this abnormality are very common in overweight and obese children. A local study assessed 46 obese children (age = 10.8, ±2.3; BMI = 27.4, ±5.1) and 44 sex- and age- matched normal weight control children (age = 11.7, ±2.1; BMI = 18, ±1.8) for obstructive sleep apnoea syndrome (OSAS) with overnight sleep studies (Wing, Hoi, Pak, et al., in press). The obese children's rate for obstructive sleep-related disordered breathing were at 10 times that of their non-obese counterparts.

Non-alcoholic steatohepatitis (NAS) or fatty liver is a well-known and potentially fatal condition in obese adults. A recent study determined the prevalence of asymptomatic NAS by ultrasonography in 84 obese children (25 girls and 59 boys with median age and body mass index (BMI) of 12.0 years [interquartile range (IR): 9.5–14.0] and 30.3 kg/m^2 (IR: 27.1–33.4) respectively) referred for medical assessment (Chan, Li, Chu, et al., personal communication). The study also determined the correlation between the severity of NAS and the degree of obesity as measured by Dual Energy X-ray Absorptiometry (DEXA) and serum biochemical abnormalities. Fasting blood samples were collected for the measurement of serum glucose, insulin and lipid profile. NAS was found in 77% of the subjects, and exhibited a significant correlation with regional fat distribution measured by DEXA at the trunk level (r = 0.25, p = 0.022), hypertriglyceridaemia (r = 0.312, p = 0.004), and index of insulin resistance (r = 0.377, $p < 0.001$). The severity of NAS was significantly correlated with insulin resistance and regional fat distribution. This study showed that this complication is very common in the more severely obese children who have been referred for medical assessment.

Joint and orthopaedic problems have been reported as complication of obesity in other countries. However no local data is available to determine the magnitude of this complication in overweight Hong Kong children.

Psychological effects of obesity in childhood may be long lasting. Local data has shown that obese children score significantly lower in their responses to questions designed to assess their self-image and their perceived physical competence. In this study of 634 children aged 8–12 years, their perceptions of specific physical competence broadly matched the evidence of specific fitness tests, showing lower scores in sports competence, coordination, flexibility and endurance relative to non-obese children, but a higher score in relation to strength (as reflected in handgrip test). Obese children did not however perceive themselves to be less healthy than non-obese children, perhaps reflecting an acceptance of the Chinese saying that "a broad heart leads to a fat body" and the widely held view that fat people tend to be happy and easy to get on with. Awareness that obesity impairs sports performance did not appear to extend to awareness that it also carries risks to health. This study also showed that obese children correctly perceived their body size, while their idea of the ideal body size was identical to that of the non-obese children. Furthermore and encouragingly, they anticipated that exercise and diet would successfully reduce their body size to normal. (Sung, unpublished data)

Although directly linking a lack of physical activity and an increased sedentary behaviour to the rapidly increasing rates of childhood obesity in Hong Kong is difficult, there is reasonable evidence that Hong Kong children are generally inactive (see chapters by Macfarlane; McManus; and Sit, Chow, & Lindner in this volume). Although increasing participation in physical activity may not by itself prevent the obesity epidemic, it is anticipated that this is likely to be a very important component. An increasing volume of local data highlights the very negative impact of childhood obesity on the health of Hong Kong children. High rates of insulin resistance, obstructive sleep apnoea syndrome and fatty liver have all been documented in obese Hong Kong children. More data is required to establish how increasing physical activity can reverse these trends and reduce these potentially serious complications.

References

Bar-Or, O., Foreyt, J., Bouchard, C., Brownell, K. D., Dietz, W. H., Ravussin, E., Salbe , A. D., Schwenger, S., St Jeor, S., & Torun, B. (1998). Physical activity, genetic, and nutritional considerations in childhood weight management. *Medicine and Science in Sports and Exercise, 30,* 2–10.

Fogelholm, M., Nuutinen, O., Pasanen, M., Myohanen, E., & Saatela, T. (1999). Parent-child relationship of physical activity patterns and obesity. *International Journal of Obesity & Related Metabolic Disorders, 23,* 1262–1268.

Fu, F. H., & Hao, X. (2002). .Physical development and lifestyle of Hong Kong secondary school students. *Preventive Medicine, 35,* 499–505.

Hernandez, B., Gortmaker, S. L., Colditz, G. A., Peterson, K. E., Laird, N. M.,

& Parra-Cabrera, S. (1999). Association of Obesity With Physical Activity, Television Programs and Other Forms of Video Viewing Among Children in Mexico City. *International Journal of Obesity & Related Metabolic Disorders, 23,* 845–854.

Hui, L. L., Nelson, E. A. S., Yu, L. M., Li, A. M., & Fok, T. F. (2003). Risk factors for childhood overweight in 6–7 year old Hong Kong children. *International Journal of Obesity, 27,* 1411–1418.

Leung, S. S., Tse, L. Y., & Leung, N. K. (1996). Growth and nutrition in Hong Kong children. *Singapore Paediatric Journal, 38,* 61–66.

Macfarlane, D. J. (1997). Some disturbing trends in the level of habitual physical activity in Hong Kong primary school children: Preliminary findings. *Hong Kong Journal of Sport Medicine and Sport Science, 5,* 42–46.

Obarzanek, E., Schreiber, G. B., Crawford, P. B., Goldman, S. R., Barrier, P. M., Frederick, M. M., & Lakatos, E. (1994). Energy intake and physical activity in relation to indexes of body fat: The National Heart, Lung, and Blood Institute Growth and Health Study. *American Journal of Clinical Nutrition, 60,* 15–22.

Sung, R. Y. T., Tong, P. C. Y, Yu, C. W., Lau, P. W. C., & Chan, J. C. N. (2003). High prevalence of insulin resistance and metabolic syndrome in overweight/obese pre-adolescent Hong Kong Chinese children 9–12 years. *Diabetes Care, 26,* 250–251.

World Health Organization (1998). Obesity: Preventing and managing the global epidemic. Geneva: Author.

Wing, Y. K., Hui, S. H., Pak, W. M., Ho, C. K., Cheung, A., Li, A. M., & Fok, T. F. (in press). A controlled study of sleep-related disordered breathing in obese children. *Archives of Diseases in Childhood.*

Woo, K. S., Chook, P., Yu, C. W., Sung, R. Y. T., et al. (2001, March). Obesity of children is associated with arterial endothelial dysfunction. Annual Scientific meeting, American College of Cardiology, Atlanta, USA.

Yu, C. W., Sung, R. Y. T., So, R., Lam, K., Nelson, E. A. S., Li, A. M. C., Yuan, Y., & Lam, P. K. W. (2002). Energy expenditure and physical activity of obese children: cross-sectional study. *Hong Kong Medical Journal, 8,* 313–317.

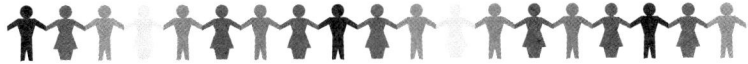

CHAPTER 8

Cardiovascular Complications Associated with Overweight and Obesity

G. Neil Thomas, Norman N. Chan, Clive S. Cockram, and Brian Tomlinson

Introduction

The rapid global rise in the prevalence of obesity has reached pandemic proportions, but more alarming, is the dramatic increase in childhood obesity (Misic, 2001). In the USA, the prevalence of obesity in children between the ages of 6 and 17 years is currently estimated at approximately 11% (Troiano & Flegal, 1998). The rising prevalence of childhood obesity has also extended to Asia, and partially explains the increase in prevalence of young-onset diabetes. Indeed, the World Health Organisation (WHO, 2000) has declared obesity as one of the top ten risk conditions in the world and one of the top five in developed nations.

Obesity is a major factor promoting the development of the disease clustering of the metabolic syndrome, namely type 2 diabetes mellitus, hypertension, dyslipidaemia and the resultant associated vascular diseases, such as coronary heart disease and stroke (World Health Organization, 2000). This is of concern as the prevalence of the metabolic syndrome in 12–19 year old Americans is high, with 4.2% having this syndrome and 28.7% of those who are obese (Cook, Weitzman, Auinger, Nguyen, & Dietz, 2003). Obesity is also associated with obstructive sleep apnoea, heart failure and some cancers, particularly colon and postmenopausal breast cancer (World Health

Organization, 2000). The morbidity and mortality from these obesity-related co-morbidities pose a serious financial burden to public health care resources. In 1998 in the USA alone, obesity has been estimated to have cost 51.6 billion US dollars (World Health Organization, 2000). The purpose of this chapter is to provide an overview of the impact of overweight and obesity on cardiovascular risk factors.

Definition of Obesity for Chinese and Asians

The practical definitions of obesity and overweight are based on body mass index (BMI), which, on a population level, is closely correlated with body fatness. BMI has two important limitations, as firstly on an individual level subjects, such as athletes with increased muscle mass can be misclassified as obese. Additionally, centrally deposited fat, particularly the visceral fat component, is more metabolically active and appears to disproportionately contribute to the risks associated with obesity. BMI does not take fat distribution into account. The BMI cut-off points for obesity are derived from statistical data from reference populations or on the excess morbidity and mortality associated with increasing body fat content. The definition for obesity in Europids is a BMI of $=25$ kg/m^2 (World Health Organization, 1998). This definition, however, does not necessarily apply to other populations or ethnic groups. Indeed, a study of more than 1500 Hong Kong Chinese clearly indicated that the risk of diabetes, hypertension, dyslipidaemia and albuminuria starts to increase at a BMI of 23 kg/m^2 (Ko, Chan, Cockram, & Woo, 1999). These data and other local findings (Figure 1) (Thomas, Tomlinson, & Critchley, 1999) support the use of obesity criteria for Hong Kong Chinese that are lower than the WHO recommendation for Europids. Similar observations have been made in other Chinese populations, including Mainland China and Singapore (He, Klag, Whelton, et al., 1994; Deurenberg-Yap, Schmidt, van Staveren, & Deurenberg, 2000). Furthermore, for a given BMI, Chinese subjects have been reported to have higher proportions of body fat than Caucasians (Deurenberg et al., 2000). These data led the WHO to suggest lower BMI cut-off points to define overweight and obesity in Asian populations (Table 1), with $=25$ kg/m^2 considered obese in these populations (World Health Organization, 2000)).

Figure 1. *Relationship between body mass index (Panel A) and waist circumference (Panel B) and the age and gender-adjusted odds ratio for Type 2 diabetes, hypertension, dyslipidaemia and a combination of the 3 disorders.* **Data show 1165 adult Hong Kong Chinese subjects with varying components of the metabolic syndrome. Analyses indicated a similar relationship for males and females between the anthropometric measures and the disorders and so the data was combined.**

A

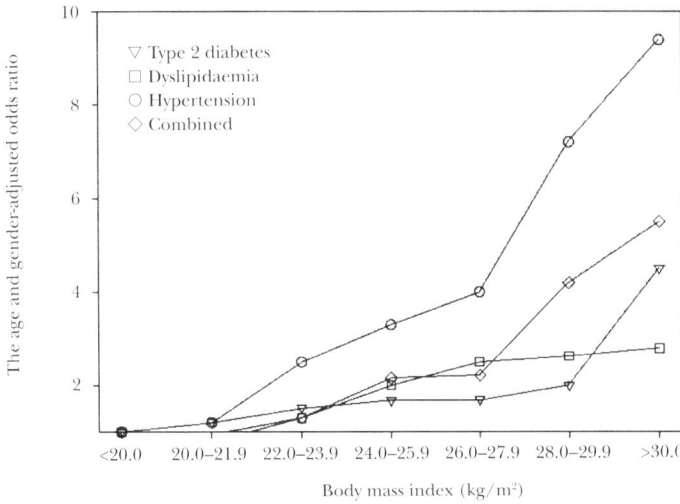

B

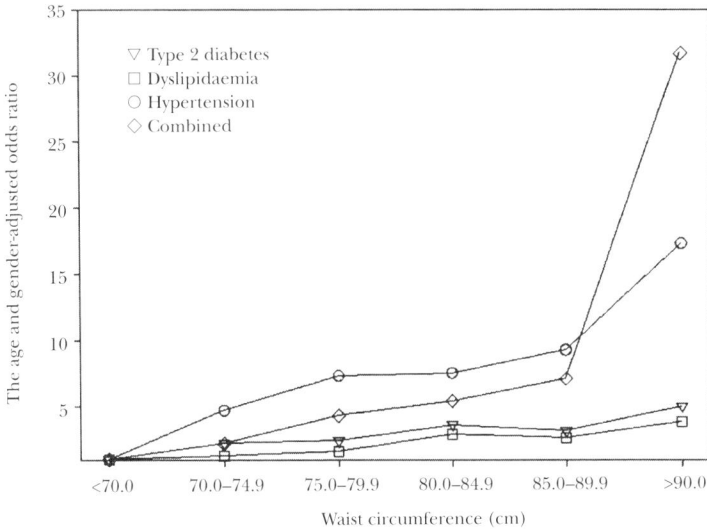

Table 1. Classification of weight by body mass index (BMI) in adult Asians

Classification	BMI (kg/m^2)	Risk of co-morbidities
Underweight	< 18.5	Low (but increased risk of other clinical problems)
Normal range	18.5–22.9	Average
Overweight	≥ 23	
At risk	23–24.9	Increased
Obese I	25–29.9	Moderate
Obese II	≥ 30	Severe

Similarly for waist circumference we have suggested in Hong Kong Chinese that an optimal level may be as low as 70cm (Thomas et al. 1999). The WHO listed provisional waist circumference-based obesity criteria as waist circumference ≥90 and ≥80 cm for Asian males and females, respectively (World Health Organization, 2000). The new guidelines for Asian populations would mean that one-third of the Hong Kong adult population would now be classified as obese with a BMI ≥25 kg/m^2 and 50% as overweight with a BMI ≥23 kg/m^2. Understanding of this concept is important since extrapolations of data from obesity studies, which were predominantly conducted in Caucasians, may need to be applied to Chinese or Asians at lower BMIs.

Childhood Obesity Predisposes to Adult Morbidity and Mortality

There is compelling evidence that childhood obesity has deleterious effects on health in adulthood (Boreham & Riddoch, 2001). Among children, physical activity and a healthy diet are associated with physiological and psychological benefits (Boreham & Riddoch, 2001). In addition, there is some evidence of tracking of behaviour and risk factors, so that excess bodyweight in children is associated with excess weight-gain in adulthood (Boreham & Riddoch, 2001; Fitzgibbon, Stolley, Dyer, VanHorn, & KauferChristoffel, 2002: Guo, Wu, Chumlea, & Roche, 2002). In the USA, a quarter of obese children have impaired glucose tolerance (Sinha, Fisch, Teague, et al., 2002) and there is increasing evidence that impaired glucose tolerance is an independent risk factor for cancer mortality (Saydah, Loria, Eberhardt, & Brancati, 2003). In a 55-year follow-up study involving over 500 children, initially aged between 13 and 18, it was found that adult men who were overweight during childhood had 2.3 times higher mortality from CHD compared to those who had normal weight during childhood (Must, Jacques, Dallal, Bajema, & Dietz, 1992). Similarly, in a 40-year follow-up study, adults who were overweight as children had 20% higher prevalence of chronic disease such as cardiovascular disease, diabetes mellitus and hypertension compared to adults who had normal weight as children (Mossberg, 1989). Furthermore, in a 37-year follow-up study of obese 18-year-old military men (BMI ≥ 31 kg/m^2), a relative risk ratio of 1.67 for mortality in obese versus nonobese group was reported and the authors found that most of the excess mortality occurred early (18–29 years) (Sonne-Holm, Sorenson, & Christiensen, 1983). These data highlight how tackling obesity early in childhood appears crucial to prevent adult morbidity and mortality from cardiovascular diseases.

Obesity and the Metabolic Syndrome

Overview of pathogenic mechanisms

Through data from epidemiological studies, it is clear that increased central abdominal fat distribution is associated with an increase in cardiovascular risk factors such as glucose intolerance and hypertension (Figure 1) (Lapidus, Bengtsson, Larsson, et al., 1984; Larsson, Svardsudd, Welin, et al., 1984; Thomas et al., 1999). The relationship between central adiposity and cardiovascular risk factors is also evident in children (Maffeis, Corciulo, Livieri, et al., 2003).

For fat accumulation to occur the energy intake from food must exceed energy expenditure from physical activity and thermogenesis, the difference being deposited as fat. Close associations have been reported between increasing levels of obesity and decreasing physical activity, as well as with increased calorific intake. Data from extreme examples, such as Sumo wrestlers, have shown that even despite very high levels of physical activity, excessive calorie intake (>5,000 compared to the 2,279 calories of the average Japanese diet) can still lead to the development of increased adiposity (Matsuzawa, Shimomura, Nakamura, Keno, & Tokunaga, 1983; Nishizawa, Akaoka, Nishida, Kawaguchi, & Hyashi, 1976). Sumo wrestlers generally have less adverse metabolic profiles than less active obese subjects, probably due to less visceral fat accumulation (Marsuzawa et al., 1983), although the profile is generally worse than age-matched healthy males (Nishizawa et al., 1976). The incidence of diabetes, and hypertension in wrestlers was 5.2, and 8.3%, respectively, which are higher than in matched controls (Nishizawa et al., 1976). However, cessation of physical activity has been associated with rapid development of visceral fat deposits (Figure 2) and subsequently metabolic disorders such as type 2 diabetes. Decreased levels of physical activity have been associated with obesity in male and female youth, and with under-weight in males (Levin, Lowry, Brown, & Dietz, 2003). Figure 2 gives an example of the high levels of visceral and subcutaneous fat in a young Type 2 diabetic female in comparison with an older healthy female.

Age-related changes further contribute to the development of cardiovascular risk in part through changes in body morphology, with reductions in lean mass and increasing body fat, which is centrally deposited. Metabolically active visceral and truncal fat depots release more non-esterified free fatty acid (FFA) that may promote peripheral and hepatic insulin resistance and the associated atherogenic lipid profiles (World Health Organization, 2000; Thomas et al., 1999). Additionally, intramyocellular lipid content has also been associated with insulin resistance in adults and youth (Weiss, Dufour, Taksali, et al., 2003). The relative hyperinsulinaemia in the obese subjects stimulates the counter-regulatory catabolic sympathoadrenal axis (Figure 3) (Landsberg, Troisi, Parker, Young, & Weiss, 1991). A similar role in the stimulation of noradrenaline secretion has also been proposed for leptin. Both BMI and waist circumference correlate closely with leptin and 24-hour urinary noradrenaline levels. A major role of noradrenaline is to stimulate thermogenesis, which is activated following feeding. Adaptive thermogenesis provides heat, but more importantly regulates energy homeostasis burning off excess calories and is a major mechanism involved in the maintenance of body weight over time. The catecholamines can mobilise energy substrates such as

Figure 2. **Magnetic resonance imaging (MRI) scans taken at L4-L5 level of A: Obese 16 year old Type 2 diabetic girl (BMI 30 kg/m², cross-sectional area of visceral 142 cm², and subcutaneous fat area 273 cm²); B: Healthy 30 year old woman (BMI 19 kg/m², cross-sectional area of visceral 15 cm², and subcutaneous fat area 128 cm²)**

A

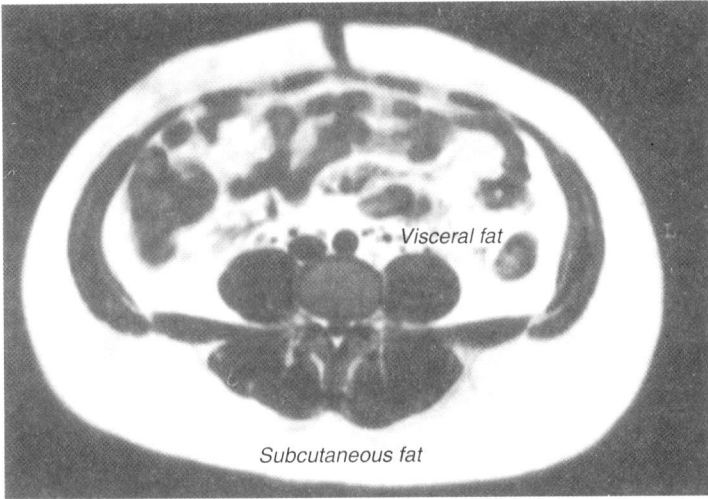

B

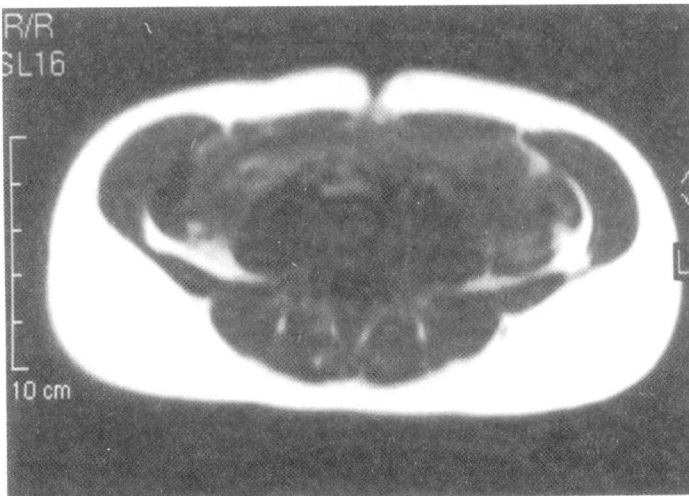

Figure 3. The complex interrelationship between obesity and hypertension with insulin resistance being the compensatory mechanism to restore energy balance and stabilise body weight.

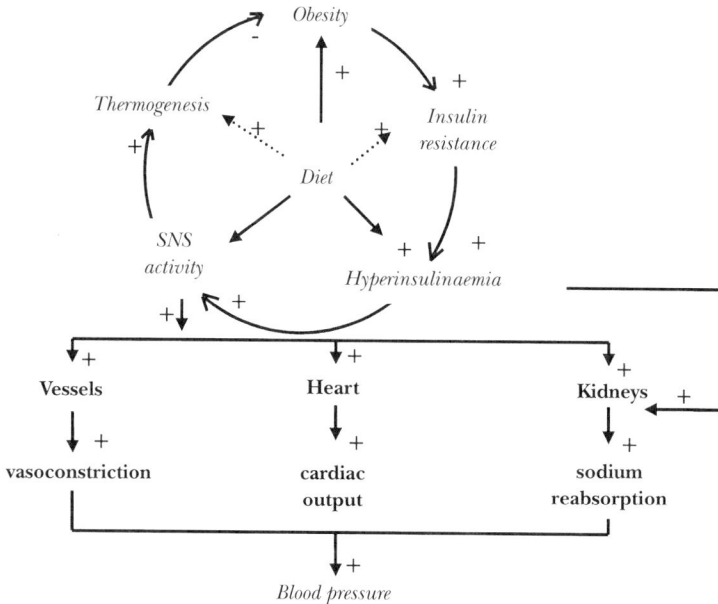

FFA or glycogen in times of energy deficiency and the former act as fuel for thermogenesis and antagonise insulin action (Landsberg, Troisi, Parker, Young, & Weiss, 1991). Increased chronic secretion of both insulin and catecholamines accentuates the insulin resistant state in obese subjects contributing further to the development of hyperglycaemia and hypertension (Reaven, Lithell, & Landsberg, 1991).

Glucose intolerance and Diabetes mellitus

The risks of developing insulin resistance and type 2 diabetes rise with increasing levels of BMI or waist circumference. In Caucasians, the scale of risk takes off exponentially above a BMI of 30 kg/m^2, but this occurs at lower levels in Chinese subjects (Figure 1). Although excess weight and obesity account for over 60% of cases of diabetes in men and over 70% of cases for women, many cases of diabetes occur in relatively lean individuals (Chan, Rimm, Colditz, Stampfer & Willet, 1994; Colditz, Willet, Rotnitzki, & Manson, 1995). This may be to some extent related to ethnic and genetic factors that determine individual susceptibility to diabetes development in relation to adiposity, and such individuals may be 'metabolically obese' (Ruderman, Chisholm, Pi-Sunyer, & Schneider, 1998). The theory that obese subjects develop diabetes through an increase in insulin resistance is supported by strong epidemiological evidence. Indeed, many obese subjects who have a normal glucose response to an oral glucose tolerance test may have hyperinsulinaemia and associated metabolic derangements such as raised triglyceride concentrations. These individuals may be considered as having 'pre-diabetes' with increased cardiovascular risk. An increased adipose tissue mass in obesity may cause insulin resistance which may result in the development of diabetes in several ways. These include enhanced lipolysis in adipose tissue leading to increased circulating FFA concentrations, deposition of triglyceride in insulin-sensitive tissue (such as muscle and liver), and humoral factors produced by adipose tissue which impair insulin action. In addition, there is some evidence that obesity may induce 'beta-cell toxicity' which may be mediated through raised FFA and triglyceride concentrations, and accumulation of islet amyloid polypeptide (Jaikaran & Clark, 2001). Other researchers have demonstrated diminished oxidative capacity of skeletal muscle for the utilisation of FFA, which may also contribute to insulin resistance (Simoneau, Colberg, Thaete, & Kelly, 1995). Our understanding of the precise mechanisms whereby obesity causes insulin resistance is far from complete and further research is required.

Hypertension

The link between obesity and hypertension is complex and incompletely understood. Obesity has been shown to predict the subsequent development of hypertension (Kannel, Brand, & Skinner, 1967). Trivial factors such as cuff artefact, excessive salt intake and other haemodynamic considerations do not account for the association between obesity and elevated blood pressure. The emergence of insulin concentrations and sympathetic nervous system (SNS) as independent risk factors contribute to the improved understanding of the underlying complex pathophysiology. The relationship between insulin and hypertension is the strongest in the obese but also exists in the non-obese , although the data in different ethnic groups are inconsistent. Much of the relationship between insulin resistance and hypertension is mediated through the obesity which causes the insulin resistance (Chan, Cheung, Lau, et al., 1996; Thomas, Critchley, Tomlinson, et al., 2000), but obesity appears to contribute to hypertension through mechanisms independent of insulin resistance (Ferrannini, Buzzigoli, Bonadonna, et al., 1987). The activity of the SNS is also closely linked to the plasma insulin concentration and SNS activity is increased in obesity and also affected by dietary changes. The alteration of SNS in turn has important effects on a several organs (heart, blood vessels and kidneys) which are involved in the regulation of arterial pressure. Fasting or a decrease in caloric intake results in a significant decrease in basal metabolic rate. In contrast, overfeeding increases metabolic heat production. These dietary-induced changes in metabolic rate are mediated through insulin and the SNS activity, and are known as dietary thermogenesis. Individuals differ in the ability for dietary thermogenesis which may have a genetic basis (Bouchard, Tremblay, Despres, et al., 1990). The interrelationship between obesity and hypertension is summarised in Figure 3. In this hypothetical model, hyperinsulinaemia serves as a compensatory mechanism in the obese subject to stabilise body weight by an increase in thermogenesis mediated through increased SNS activity and thus limits further weight gain. The increased SNS activity leads to haemodynamic effects in target organs resulting in elevated blood pressure (Landsberg et al., 1991). Accumulating research evidence supports the central role of the SNS in the pathogenesis of hypertension in obese individuals.

Several large-scale studies have shown that weight reduction is an effective intervention for hypertension in obese subjects (Langford, Blaufox, Oberman, et al., 1985; Reisin, Abel, Modan, et al., 1978). In the Dietary Approaches to Stop Hypertension (DASH), a large number of obese hypertensives were managed with withdrawal of antihypertensive therapy with concomitant sodium restriction or weight reduction, reinstitution of therapies, or no therapy (Sacks, Svetkey, Vollmer, et al., 2001). The average weight loss in the weight reduction group was 4.5 kg after 1 year. Amongst these subjects, 60% remained off medication and were normotensive, whereas only 30% in the control group were normotensive without medication. The beneficial effects of weight reduction on blood pressure were independent of gender or whether the subjects were whites or African-Americans (Langford et al., 1985). Hence a non-pharmacological approach is effective in lowering blood pressure. Similarly, our local data in Hong Kong Chinese (Tong, Lee, Chow, et al., 2002) showed that weight reduction achieved with the use of orlistat, an inhibitor of gastrointestinal lipase, resulted in significant reduction in both systolic and diastolic blood pressure in obese Chinese subjects with or without type 2 diabetes. In addition, weight reduction is accompanied by haemodynamic and cardiac structural changes (Backman, Freyschuss, Hallberg, & Melcher, 1979) resulting in reduced left ventricular stroke work leading to improved cardiac function.

Dyslipidaemia

Obesity-related dyslipidaemia is characterized by high triglyceride, low high-density lipoprotein-cholesterol (HDL-C) and often normal low-density lipoprotein-cholesterol (LDL-C) concentrations (Tomlinson, Pang, & Chan, 1998; Tomlinson & Thomas, 2003). In addition, there is a preponderance of small dense LDL particles, which further increases atherogenicity. This pattern of dyslipidaemia has been shown to be strongly associated with visceral obesity and the insulin resistance syndrome. The underlying mechanisms of these changes in lipoprotein metabolism involve increased release of free fatty acids from adipose tissue and increased triglyceride production in the liver (Tomlinson & Thomas, 2003). Triglyceride-enriched VLDL particles promote the cholesteryl ester transfer protein (CETP)-mediated exchange of triglycerides for cholesterol esters from HDL particles. The HDL particles are then rapidly catabolised by hepatic lipase and the resulting small HDL particles are rapidly removed from the circulation. In contrast the metabolism of apolipoprotein B containing particles results in small dense LDL particles which persist for longer in the circulation and are more readily oxidised resulting in an atherogenic profile. These changes were observed in the Second National Health and Nutrition Educational Survey (NHANES II), which represents a random sample of American adults within a wide range of age and socioeconomic status (Denke, Sempos, & Grundy, 1993). Weight reduction is generally associated with an improvement of this type of dyslipidaemia thereby decreasing the cardiovascular risk (Goldstein, 1992). Obese individuals appear to be less responsive to dietary approaches to cholesterol-lowering as well as to the pharmacological effects of lipid lowering drugs.

Cardiovascular disease

The clear increases in cardiovascular risk factors associated with obesity described above emphasise the likely impact on cardiovascular disease endpoints. Although the data describing the impact of BMI on vascular disease are not as strong (Curb & Marcus, 1991; Larsson, Bengtsson, Bjorntorp, et al., 1992; Rimm, Stampfer, Giovannucci, et al., 1995; Zhou, Wu, Yang, et al., 2002), central adiposity has been reported to contribute to vascular disease in a range of studies (Curb & Marcus, 1991; Rimm et al., 1995). In the Swedish Gothenburg study, CHD increased in parallel with waist-to-hip ratio, and accounted for a significant proportion of the higher CHD rates in males (Larsson et al., 1992). Similarly the Paris Prospective Study found that iliac-to-thigh ratio, another measure of central adiposity, significantly contributed to CHD mortality (Casassus, Fontbonne, Thibult, et al., 1992). The NHANES study also found that central adiposity also increased the risk of CHD mortality in Caucasian male and female subjects (Freedman, Williamson, Croft, Ballew, & Beyers, 1995), and is supported by other studies from the USA (Rimm, Stampfer, Ascherio, et al., 1993). The same study also found that obesity was an independent predictor of congestive heart failure, which was attributable to CHD in over 60% of cases (He, Ogden, Bazzano, 2001). The Honolulu Heart Program found that BMI and central adiposity contributed to CHD, whereas subscapular skinfold thickness was related to stroke (Curb & Marcus, 1991). Data from Caucasian and Oriental populations clearly show a relationship between increasing obesity and total stroke, and in particular ischaemic stroke (Zhou et al., 2002; Rexrode, Hennekens, Willett, 1997).

Conclusions

Obesity in childhood is strongly related to obesity in adulthood. Obesity, especially central adiposity, increases a range of cardiovascular risk factors that then increase the development of CHD, congestive heart failure, and stroke, particularly ischaemic stroke. As effective treatment options for obesity remain limited prevention remains the best policy. If the obesity scourge continues to increase in prevalence it will have overwhelming public health ramifications.

References

Backman, L., Freyschuss, U., Hallberg, D., & Melcher, A. (1979). Reversibility of cardiovascular changes in extreme obesity. Effects of weight reduction through jejunoileostomy. *Acta Medica Scandinavica, 205,* 367–373.

Boreham, C., & Riddoch, C. (2001). The physical activity, fitness and health of children. *Journal Sports Science, 19,* 915–929.

Bouchard, C., Tremblay, A., Despres, J. P., Nadeau, A., Lupien, P. J., Theriault, G., Dussault, J., Moorjani, S., Pinault, S., & Fournier, G. (1990). The response to long-term overfeeding in identical twins. *New England Journal of Medicine, 322,* 1477–1482.

Casassus, P., Fontbonne, A., Thibult, N., Ducimetiere, P., Richard, J. L., Claude, J. R., Warnet, J. M., Rosselin, G., & Eschwege, E. (1992). Upper-body fat distribution: a hyperinsulinaemia-independent predictor of coronary heart disease mortality. The Paris Prospective Study. *Arteriosclerosis and Thrombosis, 12,* 1387–1392.

Chan, J. C. N., Cheung, J. C. K., Lau, E. M. C., Woo, J., Chan, A. Y. W., & Cockram, C. S. (1996). The metabolic syndrome in Hong Kong Chinese. The interrelationships among its components analyzed by structural equation modeling. *Diabetes Care, 19,* 953–959.

Chan, J. M., Rimm, E. B., Colditz, G. A., Stampfer, M. J., & Willett, W. C. (1994). Obesity, fat distribution, and weight gain as risk factors for clinical diabetes in men. *Diabetes Care, 17,* 961–969.

Colditz, G. A., Willett, W. C., Rotnitzky, A., & Manson, J. E. (1995). Weight gain as a risk factor for clinical diabetes mellitus in women. *Annals of Internal Medicine, 122,* 481–486.

Cook, S., Weitzman, M., Auinger, P., Nguyen, M., & Dietz, W. H. (2003). Prevalence of a metabolic syndrome phenotype in adolescents: Findings from the Third National Health and Nutrition Examination Survey, 1988-94. *Archives of Pediatric and Adolescent Medicine, 157,* 821–827.

Curb, J. D., & Marcus, E. B. (1991). Body fat, coronary heart disease, and stroke in Japanese men. *American Journal of Clinical Nutrition, 53,* 1612S–1615S.

Denke, M. A., Sempos, C. T., Grundy, S. M. (1993). Excess body weight. An underrecognized contributor to high blood cholesterol levels in white American men. *Archives of Internal Medicine, 153,* 1093–1103.

Deurenberg-Yap, M., Schmidt, G., van Staveren, W. A., & Deurenberg, P. (2000). The paradox of low body mass index and high body fat percentage among Chinese, Malays and Indians in Singapore. *International Journal of Obesity, 24,* 1011–1017.

Ferrannini, E., Buzzigoli, G., Bonadonna, R., Giorico, M. A., Oleggini, M., Graziadei, L., Pedrinelli, R., Brandi, L., & Bevilacqua, S. (1987). Insulin resistance in essential hypertension. *New England Journal of Medicine, 317,* 350–357.

Fitzgibbon, M. L., Stolley, M. R., Dyer, A. R., VanHorn, L., & Kaufer Christoffel, K. (2002). A community-based obesity prevention program for minority children: Rationale and study design for Hip-Hop to Health. *Journal of Preventive Medicine, 34,* 289–297.

Freedman, D. S., Williamson, D. F., Croft, J. B., Ballew, C., & Byers, T. (1995). Relation of body fat distribution to ischemic heart disease. The National Health and Nutrition Examination Survey I (NHANES I) Epidemiologic Follow-up Study. *American Journal of Epidemiology, 142,* 53–63.

Goldstein, D. J. (1992). Beneficial health effects of modest weight loss. *International Journal of Obesity, 16,* 397–415.

Guo, S. S., Wu, W., Chumlea, W, C., & Roche, A. F. (2002). Predicting overweight and obesity in adulthood from body mass index values in childhood and adolescence. *American Journal of Clinical Nutrition, 76,* 653–658.

He, J., Klag, M. J., Whelton, P. K., Chen, J. Y., Qian, M. C., & He, G. Q. (1994). Body mass and blood pressure in a lean population in southwestern Chinese. *American Journal of Epidemiology, 139,* 380–389.

He, J., Ogden, L. G., Bazzano, L. A., Vupputuri, S., Loria, C., & Whelton, P. K. (2001). Risk factors for congestive heart failure in US men and women: NHANES I epidemiologic follow-up study. *Archives of Internal Medicine, 161*, 996–1002.

Jaikaran, E. T., & Clark, A. (2001). Islet amyloid and type 2 diabetes: From molecular misfolding to islet pathophysiology. *Biochimica & Biophysica Acta, 1537*, 179–203.

Kannel, W. B., Brand, N., Skinner Jr, J. J., Dawber, T. R., & McNamara P. M. (1967). The relation of adiposity to blood pressure and development of hypertension. *Annals of Internal Medicine, 67*, 48–59.

Ko, G. T. C, Chan, J. C. N., Cockram, C. S., & Woo, J. (1999). Prediction of hypertension, diabetes, dyslipidaemia or albuminuria using simple anthropometric indexes in Hong Kong Chinese. *International Journal of Obesity, 23*, 1136–1142.

Landsberg, L., Troisi, R., Parker, D., Young, J. B., & Weiss, S. T. (1991). Obesity, blood pressure, and the sympathetic nervous system. *Annals of Epidemiology, 1*, 295–303.

Langford, H. G., Blaufox, M. D., Oberman, A., Hawkins, C. M., Curb, J. D., Cutter, G. R., Wassertheil-Smoller, S., Pressel, S., Babcock, C., Abernethy, J. Df, et al. (1985). Dietary therapy slows the return of hypertension after stopping prolonged medication. *Journal of the American Medical Association, 253*, 657–664.

Lapidus, L., Bengtsson, C., Larsson, B., Penner, K., Rybo, E., & Sjostrom, L. (1984). Distribution of adipose tissue and risk of cardiovascular disease and death: a 12-year follow-up of participants in the population study of women in Gothenburg, Sweden. *British Medical Journal, 289*, 1257–1261.

Larsson, B., Bengtsson, C., Bjorntorp, P., Lapidus, L., Sjostrom, L., Svardsudd, K., Tibblin, G., Wedel, H., Welin, L., & Wilhelmsen, L. (1992). Is abdominal body fat distribution a major explanation for the sex difference in the incidence of myocardial infarction? The study of men born in 1913 and the study of women, Goteborg, Sweden. *American Journal of Epidemiology, 135*, 266–273.

Larsson, B., Svardsudd, K., Welin, L., Wilhelmsen, L., Bjorntorp, P., & Tibblin, G. (1984). Abdominal adipose tissue distribution, obesity, and risk of cardiovascular disease and death: a 13-year follow-up of participants in the Study of Men Born in 1913. *British Medical Journal, 288*, 1401–1404.

Levin, S., Lowry, R., Brown, D. R., & Dietz, W. H. (2003). Physical activity and body mass index among US adolescents: Youth risk behavior survey, 1999. *Archives of Pediatric and Adolescent Medicine, 157*, 816–820.

Maffeis, C., Corciulo, N., Livieri, C., Rabbone, I., Trifiro, G., Falorni, A., Guerraggio, L., Peverelli, P., Cuccarolo, G., Bergamaschi, G., Di Pietro, M., & Grezzani, A. (2003). Waist circumference as a predictor of cardiovascular and metabolic risk factors in obese girls. *European Journal of Clinical Nutrition, 57*, 566–572.

Matsuzawa, Y., Shimomura, I., Nakamura, T., Keno, Y., & Tokunaga, K. (1983). Pathophysiology and pathogenesis of visceral fat obesity. *Annals of the New York Academy of Scienes, 676*, 270–278.

Micic, D. (2001). Obesity in children and adolescents-a new epidemic? Consequences in adult life. *Journal of Pediatric Endocrinology and Metabolism, 14*, 1345–1352; discussion 1365.

Mossberg, H. O. (1989). 40-year follow-up of overweight children. *The Lancet, 2*, 491–493.

Must, A., Jacques, P. F., Dallal, G. E., Bajema, C. J., & Dietz, W. H. (1992). Long-term morbidity and mortality of overweight adolescents. A follow-up of the Harvard Growth Study of 1922 to 1935. *New England Journal of Medicine, 327*, 1350–1355.

Nishizawa, T., Akaoka, I., Nishida, Y., Kawaguchi, Y., & Hayashi, E. (1976). Some factors related to obesity in the Japanese sumo wrestler. *American Journal of Clinical Nutrition, 29*, 1167–1174.

Reaven, G. M., Lithell, H., & Landsberg, L. (1996). Hypertension and associated metabolic abnormalities - the role of insulin resistance and the sympathoadrenal system. *New England Journal of Medicine, 334*, 374–381.

Rexrode, K. M., Hennekens, C. H., Willett, W. C., Colditz, G. A., Stampfer, M. J., Rich-Edwards, J. W., Speizer, F. E., & Manson, J. E. (1997). A prospective study of body mass index, weight change, and risk of stroke in women. *Journal of the American Medical Association, 277*, 1539–1545.

Reisin, E., Abel, R., Modan, M., Silverberg, D. S., Eliahou, H. E., & Modan, B. (1978). Effect of weight loss without salt restriction on the reduction of blood pressure in overweight hypertensive patients. *New England Journal of Medicine, 298*, 1–6.

Rimm, E. B., Stampfer, M. J., Ascherio, A., Giovannucci, E., Colditz, G. A., & Willett, W. C. (1993). Vitamin E consumption and the risk of coronary disease in men. *New England Journal of Medicine, 328*, 1450–1456.

Rimm, E. B., Stampfer, M. J., Giovannucci, E., Ascherio, A., Spiegelman, D.,

Colditz, G. A., & Willett, W. C. (1995). Body size and fat distribution as predictors of coronary heart disease among middle-aged and older US men. *American Journal of Epidemiology, 141,* 1117–1127.

Sacks, F. M., Svetkey, L. P., Vollmer,W. M., Appel, L. J., Bray, G. A., Harsha, D., Obarzanek, E., Conlin, P. R., Miller, E. R., Simons-Morton, D. G., Karanja, N., & Lin, P. H. (2001). Effects on blood pressure of reduced dietary sodium and the Dietary Approaches to Stop Hypertension (DASH) diet. DASH-Sodium Collaborative Research Group. *New England Journal of Medicine,* 344, 3–10.

Saydah, S. H., Loria, C. M., Eberhardt, M. S., & Brancati, F. L. (1992). Abnormal glucose tolerance and the risk of cancer death in the United States. *American Journal of Epidemiology, 157,* 1092–1100.

Simoneau, J. A., Colberg, S. R., Thaete, F. L., & Kelley, D. E. (1995). Skeletal muscle glycolytic and oxidative enzyme capacities are determinants of insulin sensitivity and muscle composition in obese women. *FASEB Journal, 9,* 273–278.

Sinha, R., Fisch, G., Teague, B., Tamborlane, W. V., Banyas, B., Allen, K., Savoye, M., Riege,r V., Taksali, S., Barbetta, G., Sherwin, R. S., & Caprio, S. (2002). Prevalence of impaired glucose tolerance among children and adolescents with marked obesity. *New England Journal of Medicine, 346,* 802–810.

Sonne-Holm, S., Sorensen, T. I., & Christensen, U. (1983). Risk of early death in extremely overweight young men. *British Medical Journal, 287,* 795–797.

Ruderman, N., Chisholm, D., Pi-Sunyer, X., & Schneider, S. (1998). The metabolically obese, normal-weight individual revisited. *Diabetes, 47,* 699–713.

Thomas, G. N., Critchley, J. A., Tomlinson, B., Anderson, P. J., Lee, Z. S., & Chan, J. C. (2000). Obesity, independent of insulin resistance, is a major determinant of blood pressure in normoglycaemic Hong Kong Chinese. *Metabolism, 49,* 1523–1528.

Thomas, G. N., Tomlinson, B., & Critchley, J. A. (1999). Guidelines for healthy weight [letter]. *New England Journal of Medicine, 341,* 2097–2098.

Tomlinson, B., Pang, C. C. P., & Chan, P. (1998). Hyperlipidaemia in Chinese populations. *Hospital Medicine, 59,* 549–552.

Tomlinson, B., & Thomas, G. N. (2003). Hyperlipidemia. In J. J. Y. Sung, L. S. K. Wong, P. K. T. Li, J. Sanderson, & T. C. Y. Kwok (Eds.). *Principles and practice of clinical medicine in Asia: Treating the Asian patient* (pp. 526–538). Hong Kong: Lippincott, Williams and Wilkins.

Tong, P. C., Lee, Z. S., Sea, M. M., Chow, C. C., Ko, G. T., Chan, W. B., So, W. Yy, Ma, R. C., Ozaki, R., Woo, J., Cockram, C. S., & Chan, J. C. (2002). The effect of orlistat-induced weight loss, without concomitant hypocaloric diet, on cardiovascular risk factors and insulin sensitivity in young obese Chinese subjects with or without type 2 diabetes. *Archives of Internal Medicine, 162,* 2428–2435.

Troiano, R. P., & Flegal, K. M. (1998). Overweight children and adolescents: description, epidemiology, and demographics. *Pediatrics, 101,* 497–504.

Weiss, R., Dufour, S., Taksali, S. E., Tamborlane, W. V., Petersen, K. F., Bonadonna, R. C., Boselli, L., Barbetta, G., Allen, K., Rife, F., Savoye, M., Dziura, J., Sherwin, R., Shulman, G. I., & Caprio, S. (2003). Prediabetes in obese youth: a syndrome of impaired glucose tolerance, severe insulin resistance, and altered myocellular and abdominal fat partitioning. *The Lancet, 362,* 951–957.

World Health Organization (1998). *Obesity: Preventing and managing the global epidemic.* Geneva: Author.

World Health Organization (2001). *The Asia-Pacific perspective: Redefining obesity and its treatment.* Canberra: Health Communications Australia.

Zhou, B., Wu, Y., Yang, J., Li, Y., Zhang, H., & Zhao, L. (2002). Overweight is an independent risk factor for cardiovascular disease in Chinese populations. *Obesity Review, 3,* 147–156.

PART IV

Factors in Physical Activity Participation

This section of the book further examines possible factors affecting physical activity participation in Hong Kong. Several earlier chapters have speculated on the roles such factors may play (e. g., Macfarlane in Chapter 4, McManus in Chapter 5, and Sit, Chow and Lindner in Chapter 6), but a more comprehensive inspection is presented here.

In Chapter 9, Cecilia Au presents the findings from the quantitative aspect of her investigation into the role of socializing agents as perceived by Hong Kong youth. The influencing role of the family was perceived lower than those of friends and the physical education teacher. Parental encouragement was particularly low in respondents with infrequent or rare participation, confirming findings presented in Chapter 6. Chinese culture and Confucian philosophy were regarded explanatory for the findings.

David Johns analyses the role of school physical education in physical activity participation by Hong Kong children in Chapter 10, and discusses government policies, curriculum issues, current practices and the status of the subject and its teachers. The school is theoretically the ideal and perhaps the only place to instill positive habits, but a major change in the physical education curriculum would be required if it is to fulfil this role. Bringing curriculum innovations to the practitioners and having them implement these is problematic to such an extent that ideas may fade before they can be put into practice. Johns presents his thoughts on the nature of the ideal physical education curriculum and how it could be implemented.

In the next chapter David Johns and Patricia Vertinsky look at a broader range of influences on health-related activity. The interaction of the Hong Kong physical environment with social, cultural and psychological factors creates a unique but unfavourable context for habitual physical activity. The authors analyze such factors as climate, space restrictions, limited facilities, study/work focus and Chinese culture and traditions in their effort to paint the background for the lack of physical activity participation in Hong Kong children and youth.

CHAPTER *9*

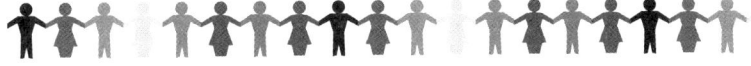

The Perceived Influence of Socialising Agents on Hong Kong Youth's Entry into Sports Participation

Cecilia King Fan Au

Introduction

Numerous studies have demonstrated that physically active children are more likely to grow up to be active adults (Dennison, Straus, Mellits, & Charney, 1988; Engstrom, 1986; Jeziorski, 1994; Sofranko & Nolan, 1972; Yang, Telama, & Laakso, 1996; Yoesting & Burkhead, 1973). These studies implied that if children are exposed to sports in their younger years, they will adopt the habit of sport participation and will most likely continue participating in sport in their adulthood. Then, the important question is, how do children become involved in sports? As Digel (1995) has stated, children are not born with but socialised into different values and behaviours and in this case, into physical activity or sport participation. The concept of socialisation is understood as a social process whereby individuals in society absorb particular values, standards, and beliefs current or more dominant in that society (Coakley, 1987, 1998). Everyone in a society learns through agents of socialisation, such as school, home, the mass media, etc., but the outcomes of social learning are not easily accounted for nor are they predictable. Nevertheless, socialisation continues to be a useful concept in gaining a better understanding of the nature of the agents who assist the individual in the acquisition of values and beliefs.

According to Kenyon and McPherson (1973, cited by Butcher, 1983) and Bandura (1977, cited by Higginson, 1985) and Dyck (2003), the process of socialisation into sport participation depends on the personal attributes, the influence of socialising agents such as parents, coaches and peers, and whether the opportunities to play sport are available. McPherson and Brown (1980, cited in Smoll, Magill, & Ash, 1988, p. 268) and Stroot (2002) concluded quite similarly that the three main elements of the socialisation process include socialising agents, or sources of social support, who serve as role models; various social environments (e.g., home, school, class, gymnasium, neighbour-hood), which provide the opportunity and encouragement for activity; and role learners, who possess a wide variety of ascribed and achieved personal attributes (e.g., personality traits, attitudes, motivation, values, motor ability, race, ethnicity, gender). These studies were based on a functionalist theory that assumed that a process of internalization takes place in a range of circumstances and conditions rendering the child socialized to one degree or another.

Although modern sociologists have questioned these assumptions, and are now in favour of conducting qualitative research to investigate into sport experience in people's lives (Coakley, 2001), it is still useful to obtain a broad picture of populations that have not been examined. The initial concepts developed to conduct early studies still have relevance today. For example, these studies showed that socialising agents are among the key elements in the initial stage influencing sports participation. They either exert positive, implying encourage-ment, or negative, implying discouragement of participation, and the effect can be observed in the later stages of child development. The early studies by Greendorfer, (1977), Higginson (1985), and Snyder and Spreitzer (1978) have all shown that a positive influence by the agent will yield a positive response from the recipient. Thus, if physical education and sport activities are valued in a society, the younger generation should hold similar values and become socialised into them.

The chapter is based on a study (Au, 1998) conducted to investigate to what extent socialising agents are perceived by students to have influenced them to engage in sports prior to entering university. This chapter examines the agents that exert positive or negative influences on young people and will provide an alternative explanation to those expressed by other authors in this section who have examined the environmental and social influences that are likely to affect participation.

Most of the published research on socialising agents (Coakley, 1987, 2001; Greendorfer, 1977; Greendorfer & Lewko, 1978; Higginson, 1985; Jeziorski, 1994; Smith, 1979; Snyder & Spreitzer, 1976a, 1978; Stroot, 2002; Wold & Anderssen, 1992) has been based on the study of populations from predominantly Western cultural backgrounds in countries such as United Kingdom, Canada, Sweden and the USA. With the exception of Yamaguchi (1984), who compared Japanese and Canadian adolescent socialisation into sport, no research has examined other Asian populations. Furthermore, the published research has primarily focused on competitive elite athletes or intercollegiate players participating in sports. Consequently, there remains a dearth of research investigating physical activity participation for health, fitness and enjoyment. The need to investigate the situation in Hong Kong is particularly salient considering the concern expressed over low participation rates in physical activity in Hong Kong children and youth (e.g., Lindner, 1998; Macfarlane, 1997; McManus & Armstrong, 1996).

Investigating the Case of Hong Kong Youth

This study examined the perceived influence of socialising agents with respect to sports participation among youths of Hong Kong in order to understand how students perceived their families, peer groups, coaches, schools, religious groups and the media as a positive (encouraging) or negative (discouraging) influence on their participation. In order to conduct this study, I surveyed 3,151 new entrants to the University of Hong Kong (HKU) in the year 1996 comprising 1,454 males and 1,697 females. Although there were a number of mature and graduate students among the respondents, the mean age was 21.5 years and approximately 88% of the respondents were mostly within the age range of 16–21 years. Although there was no formal investigation conducted regarding the ethnicity of the students who came from all parts of Hong Kong, 87 % were born in Hong Kong and 11% were from China (Office of Student Affairs, 1995, 1996). It is recognized that the sample comprised a special segment of the population and thus is not representative of all youth in Hong Kong.

Questions on socializing agents were embedded in a four part questionnaire in which respondents were asked to select and indicate on a 5-point scale the strength of their selection as either 'encouraged' or 'discouraged' for each of the 13 socializing agents. Past participation in physical activity was measured in a question that required the respondent to indicate the frequency of their participation on a scale from 0 (seldom or never) to 5 (almost daily). The respondents were recorded into four frequency of participation groups: "Seldom or Never"(O or 1); "Occasional" (2), "Regular" (3), and "Frequent" (4 or 5). The data were entered and analysed using "Statview" statistic software. Multivariate ANOVA with repeated measurements was used to analyse the strength of the perceived influences for each agency group and individual agents within the groups, and for comparison of participation frequency groups. Chi-square was used to determine whether there were significant differences between males and females with regard to the percentages of them indicating certain socialising agents as more influential.

Results

I found that in general the majority of the respondents perceived all agents to be encouraging towards sport participation but certain agents were more strongly associated with encouragement while others were ranked less so (Table 1). For example, male students selected their male friends most often as a positive influence on their participation, followed by the physical education teacher and parents, whereas females selected female friends, followed by the physical education teacher and then male friends and siblings. Relatively few indicated that the agents had been a hindrance to their participation.

Table 1 identifies the agents that were perceived as positively or negatively influential in their participation in physical activity. However, these proportions do not reflect the degree to which the agents were perceived as positive or negative forces and therefore may change when the weighting is considered. When strength and weakness of endorsement was considered, an ANOVA showed that both genders

Table 1. Percentages of male and female respondents perceiving socialising agents as encouraging or discouraging

Agent	Males (N = 1,154)			Females (N = 1,697)		
	Rank	Enc*	Disc**	Rank	Enc*	Disc**
Father	3	72	3	5	76	4.5
Mother	4	72	5	6	76	6
Siblings	6	68	1	3	76	1.5
M. Friends	1	79	0.5	3	76	1.5
F. Friends	5	70	1.5	1	82	2.5
Coach	12	56	0.5	12	62	1.5
School Tradition	7	68	5	9	70	8.5
School Principal	11	59	3.5	11	65	4.5
PE Teacher	2	72	2	2	79	2.5
Religion	13	39	1	13	46	2
Newspapers	10	59	1	10	66	1
Television	8	67	0.5	7	72	1.5
Magazines	9	66	0.5	8	70	1

* Enc = Encourage   ** Dis = Discourage

Note: remaining percentages pertain to those who did not select either
    Encourage or Discourage.

rated significant others, higher than other groups, while females rated the family, significant others and media groups lower than the males. Apparently, the assumption that the family is the most important influence on activity participation was not supported in this study due perhaps to the age of the respondents. One can conclude that as children become adolescents they will be more likely to name peers rather than their family members as being instrumental in influencing physical activity behaviours (Higginson, 1985; Patriksson, 1981) and it may also reflect that Chinese parental involvement in physical activity decreases with age.

Table 2 shows that significant others as a group have the highest average means among the four main socialising agency groups. This is consistent with the earlier findings by Snyder and Spreitzer (1976a, 1976b, 1978), Greendorfer (1977), Greendorfer, Pellegrini, and Blinde (1985), Higginson (1985), Coakley (1987), Lewko and Greendorfer (1988), Sohi and Singh (1986), and Wold and Anderssen

Table 2. **Ranks, means and standard deviations of the four socialising
          agents groups by gender**

Agency Group	Males			Females		
	Rank	Mean	SD	Rank	Mean	SD
Family	2	2.18	1.08	3	2.08	1.14
Significant Others	1	2.43	0.85	1	2.22	0.97
School	3	2.13	1.17	2	2.12	1.19
Media	4	2.02	0.81	4	1.88	0.87

(1992) who also found that significant others is aptly named because
the influence of this group is clearly shown. The place of the specific
agents within the four groups will be examined next.

Individual socializing agents

Same-sex friends were shown to be significantly more influential for
males than the other agents in the significant others group. Although
male respondents ranked agents consistently higher than females and
coaches as more important than the females did, females ranked the
PE teacher higher than their females friends and siblings. The PE
teacher was considered by both males and females to be influential
and was rated high by both genders. Religion was rated significantly
lower as a socializing force than the other three agents by both males
and females. Although there were no differences in ratings among
television, magazines and newspapers for the females, the males rated
the media agents significantly higher than the females , and television
much higher than newspapers. Other than looking at the agents in
their own group, comparing the collective effect of all the socialising
agents, it was found that males ranked their male friends, PE teachers
and coaches highest, while females ranked the PE teacher, their female
friends and their siblings as the most influential. When the gender
categories are combined, not surprisingly, male friends and PE teachers
were significantly more influential than school principals or religion.

Even though it is not the intention of this study to expressly discuss
one gender over another, the result has manifested some prominent
gender issues of female sport participation. Similar to many studies

Table 3. Ranks, means and standard deviations of socializing agents by gender

Agent	Males			Females		
	Rank	Mean	SD	Rank	Mean	SD
Father	7	2.18	1.32	6	2.01	1.28
Mother	8	2.12	1.34	6	2.01	1.38
Siblings	5	2.25	1.08	3	2.22	1.21
M. Friends	1	2.70	1.00	4	2.17	1.20
F. Friends	4	2.26	1.14	2	2.35	1.19
Coach	3	2.34	1.07	5	2.15	1.19
School Tradition	10	2.04	1.60	11	1.94	1.64
School Principal	12	1.91	1.38	12	1.88	1.32
PE Teacher	2	2.43	1.32	1	2.54	1.24
Religion	13	1.77	1.03	13	1.64	1.08
Newspapers	11	2.00	1.00	9	1.95	1.03
Television	6	2.18	1.02	9	1.95	1.12
Magazines	8	2.12	0.95	8	1.96	1.08

on women participation (Greendorfer, 1992; Jeziorski, 1994; Kew, 1997; Stroot, 2001; Weistart, 2001), the frequency of female participation in sports is significantly lower as compared to male participation. More females than males reported that they were discouraged from participating directly by their mothers and indirectly through a school ethos that condones passivity in females rather than encouraging them to be active. Similar to Humberstone's (2002) findings male domination of the school playground in Hong Kong is also a contributing factor to females' perceived lack of opportunity in school. These evidences imply that gender stereotyping within the school and family agencies may have caused the marginalization of sport participation among Hong Kong females.

Past participation in sports

One of the aspects of the study that is particularly relevant to this section of the book, examined the effect of socialization on habitual physical activity. On close examination it was found that of the male respondents 16% were frequently active, 47% indicated they were regularly active, and 37% were inactive or only occasionally engaged in physical activities. For the females these figures were 8%, 31% and 62% respectively and show a close relationship to the rates presented by Sit, Chow and Lindner in Chapter 6. I was able to show that the high percentage of individuals who perceived various agents to be influential was not reflected in the numbers who exercised regularly. Clearly, the large number of students who do not participate regularly, even though they perceived to have been positively encouraged, demonstrate that such encouragement is not always internalized and translated into physical activity. Moreover, when parental and school encouragement is perceived to be weak and discouragement high, respondents are much more likely to be less active than the other three frequency groups.

Linking agents and participation

Generally, there is a relationship between participation rates and how respondents perceived the level of agent encouragement. There is a clear increase in ratings with increase in sports participation. Males who do not participate have low rating of the perceived encouragement of sports participation by agents. In contrast, respondents who participated more often reported higher rating of perceived agent encouragement. Male friends were the strongest-rated agents in all frequency groups and the PE teacher was second in all but the frequent participation group, where (s)he was fourth highest. School tradition increased in importance with increasing frequency of participation. Responses for females were similar, showing that individuals with low participation levels rated the socialising agents much lower in their encouragement than the other groups with an increase in ratings coinciding with an increase in participation frequency. The PE teacher and the female friends were rated highest, in that order, in each frequency group, the perceived influence of the family group increased and that of television and magazines decreased with increasing participation frequency.

Discussion

The results report the extent of the effect that socializing agents are perceived to have had on beginning sports participation by students entering university. It was conjectured that if students experience or perceive encouragement to participate in physical activity, they actually will, and the stronger the encouragement, the higher the frequency of participation. By the same token, if students are being negatively socialised with discouragement to become involved in physical activity, they will not be inclined to participate, and the stronger the discourage-ment, the lower participation will it be. From what I found, it is clear that the majority of students perceived all the agents to be encouraging or positive towards sports participation. The results also indicate that the stronger or more positive the encouragement the higher the frequency in participation, thus showing that a process of internaliza-tion may account for the rates of involvement. Conversely, when students received negative or weak encouragement they showed little or no interest in participation. Such findings have been reported in the literature by Snyder and Spreitzer (1978) who reported that girls who were non-participants in sports and music were characterised by a low degree of perceived parental encouragement for either extra-curricular activity.

Apart from the socialising agents, there are of course many other factors that are thought to influence participation in physical activity. As mentioned in Chapters 4 and 8, social and environmental factors such as the provision and quality of equipment and facilities, the quality of physical education programming in addition to parental support are possible influential factors in the decision to participate in physical activity. The personal attributes, the availability of opportunities, sufficient facilities, and suitable environment are all important factors that in combination with significant social influences determine the degree and direction to which young people are socialized (Sewell, 1963, cited in McPherson et al., 1989).

Cultural factors affecting socialization

Apart from the factors that have already been identified, there are additional considerations that are particularly unique to the Chinese culture. One of the most discussed issues in Chinese education is the concern and indoctrination of students to study (Postiglione & Lee,

1995). This dedication to academic learning is characterized by its intolerance of behaviours and habits that are thought to inhibit learning. Physical activities are viewed with disdain when they are perceived to compete with time and attention for study. In addition, Hong Kong is an instrumental culture that places little value on pursuits that have no direct relationship to success which is understood in Chinese society to be a means of selection for further educational and career opportunities (Gow, Balla, Kember, & Hau, 1996). Success in public examinations is of utmost importance and is a widely acclaimed act of aggregation that is celebrated by the students, teachers and parents. Therefore, sport and physical activity is perceived to have no bearing on academic success or entry into university and is marginalized and trivialized in the school curriculum (Johns & Dimmock, 1999).

The results reflect these attitudes towards physical activity as seen in relatively lower ratings of school tradition and the school principal as perceived agents of socialization. The emphasis on academic study rather than physical activity is related to the fierce competition for university places in Hong Kong in which qualifications have been limited to academic standing only. Only recently has special consideration been given to students who have demonstrated a high degree of expertise in music, art and sport. The result of the recent liberalization of qualifications is unknown as many concerned parents continue to restrict their children's participation in less valid academic subjects in the hope that they will devote more time preparing for public examination and later the University entrance examination. This over-concern for time to study was reported in Lindner's study (1995) in which over 50% of the University entrants claimed the need to study as one of the reasons for not participating in sport or physical activities (Lindner, 1995).

Confucian influences

There are also cultural aspects to the socialisation into the sport process and the age old attitudes towards child rearing and the internalization of behaviours that were deemed particularly appropriate for upper class upbringing. For centuries, Chinese have been guided by the principles of Confucius in the upbringing and socialisation of the children. Confucian families of the gentry placed great emphasis on composed, reverential behaviour that focused on a disposition of solemnity, self-control, and personal restraint of physical activity. Guidelines for parents on family education written after the fourteenth century emphasise that the behaviour of children should ensure "no leaping, arguing, joking, slouching, or using vulgar language" All "violent exercise was discouraged, and a boy was taught that the more dignified and grave his deportment, the greater approbation he would receive from his elders" (Dardess, 1991, cited in Wu, 1996, p. 146).

The extent to which modern Hong Kong families adhere to these guiding principles is difficult to assess. Nevertheless, vestiges of Confucianism remain and are particularly noticeable in the intolerance and trivialization of physical activity and the accommodation and valourisation of study of valid subjects (Morris, 1995) in the school curriculum. Some neo-Confucian scholars reflect these attitudes in the way they encouraged parents and teachers to direct the child away from engaging in silly behaviour (Dardess, 1991, cited in Wu, 1996). However, under the assumption that children are engaged in worthy educational pursuits as long as they are in front of a computer, parents tolerate the passive hours spent alone.

Similar to the patterns of family life in other modern societies, Hong Kong fathers are less concerned with the process than the outcome, while mothers, who also work, are concerned with both. In Hong Kong this is expressed in terms of the Confucian ethic in which the status ascribed to parents and in particular the father whose role as head of the family is to make the rules and maintain them "irrespective of whether the demands or requests at times seem unreasonable" (Gow et al., 1996, p.114). The role of the mother is to obey her husband by ensuring that children are fed, clothed, prepared for school, and that they fulfill the over emphasized demands for homework. Perhaps this is why the father was not perceived to be a major agent on the socialization process.

In the Chinese culture of Hong Kong, children are said to be brought up in a very disciplined environment in which they have to listen to their parents and be obedient and respectful to their elders. A principle of filial piety, that justifies absolute authority on the basis of generational seniority, "has served as a guiding principle governing general Chinese patterns of socialisation, as well as specific rules of intergenerational conduct, applicable throughout the length of one's life span" (Ho, 1987, p. 155). It can be argued that filial piety is a traditional process of socialisation of the child in which training for obedience, for proper conduct, impulse control, and acceptance of social obligations are upheld and reinforced , while independence, assertiveness, and creativity de-emphasised (Wu, 1996). However, while filial piety may explain the way some adolescents have matured into ideal adults, it does not explain why others have been less successful leaving us to speculate further as to the mechanisms that are currently at work in nurturing our children into adulthood.

Conclusion

Hong Kong youth are similar to those young people who have been the subject of examination of socialization in other countries. In general, all the usual socialising agents found in previous studies are also common in the socialization process into sports of Hong Kong youth. For example, it is found that male friends were perceived by the male students as the most influential agent while female students perceived their PE teachers to be the most influential agent for sports participation. These findings would suggest that Hong Kong society is not very different from other societies. However, as others have suggested, the youth population is subjected to some unique influences that can be attributed to the more sedentary lifestyles that young people in Hong Kong tend to live.

While socialisation as a way of understanding the process of internalizing social and cultural expectations is useful in accounting for much of what we see in our children, we should not accept that all societies are similar. I have tried to show in discussing the outcomes of my study that the role of specific cultural and social influences may have their own unique influences on a society thus inscribing the society with its own distinctiveness and individuality. For example, one could argue that the Confucian ethic and the role of filial piety is unique but can be identified using the model of internalization as an effective process that teaches children the social values and beliefs that are appropriate for that society. In any efforts to change the physical activity attitudes and habits of Hong Kong youth it would do well to bear in mind that this region reflects the dominant developed nations of the world in terms of political, economic and popular culture, but still remains a unique Chinese culture in other respects.

References

Au, C. K. F. (1998). *The perceived influence of socializing agents on Hong Kong youth's entry into sports participation.* Unpublished M.Sc. Thesis, The University of Leicester.

Butcher, J. (1983). Socialization of adolescent girls into physical activity. *Adolescence, 18,* 753–766.

Coakley, J. J. (1987). Children and the sport socialization process. *Advances in Paediatrics, 2,* 43–60.

Coakley, J. J. (1998). *Sport in society: Issues and controversies* (6th edition). Boston, MA: McGraw-Hill.

Coakley, J. J. (2001). *Sport in society: Issues and controversies* (7th edition). New York: McGraw-Hill Higher Education.

Dardess, J. (1991). Childhood in pre-modern China. In J. M. Hawes, M. Joseph, & N. R. Hiner (Eds.), *Childhood in historical and comparative perspective* (pp. 71–94), New York: Greenwood.

Dennison, B. A., Straus, J. H., Mellits, E. D., & Charney, E. (1988). Childhood physical fitness test: Predictor of adult physical fitness levels? *Pediatrics, 82,* 324–330.

Digel, H. (1995). Sport in a changing society. *International Council of Sports Science and Physical Education: Sport Science Studies, Volume 7.*

Dyck, N. (2003). Embodying success: identity and performance in children's sport. In N. Dyck & E. P. Archetti (Eds.), *Sport, dance and embodied identities* (pp. 55–73). New York: Berg.

Engstrom, L. M. (1986). The process of socialization into keep-fit activities. *Scandinavian Journal of Sports Science, 8,* 89–97.

Gow, L., Balla, J., Kember, D., & Hau, K. T. (1996). The learning approach of Chinese people: A function of socialization processes and the context of learning? In M. H. Bond (Ed.), *The handbook of Chinese psychology* (pp. 109–123). Hong Kong: Oxford University Press.

Greendorfer, S. (1977). Role of socializing agents in female sport involvement. *Research Quarterly, 48,* 304–310.

Greendorfer, S. L. (1992). Differences in childhood socialization influences of women involved in sport and women not involved in sport. In A. Yiannakis & S. L. Greendorfer (Eds.), *Applied sociology of sport* (pp. 111–124), Champaign, IL: Human Kinetics.

Greendorfer, S., & Lewko, J. (1978). Role of family members in sport socialization of children. *Research Quarterly, 49,* 146–152.

Greendorfer, S., Pellegrini, A. M., & Blinde, E. M. (1985). *Gender differences in American and Brazilian children's socialization into sport.* Illinois Sociological Association.

Higginson, D. C. (1985). The influence of socializing agents in the female sport-participation process. *Adolescence, 20,* 73–82.

Ho, D. Y. F. (1989). Continuity and variation in Chinese patterns of socialization. *Journal of Marriage and the Family, 51,* 149–163.

Humberstone, B. (2002). Femininity, masculinity and difference: what's wrong with a sarong? In A. Laker (Ed.), *The sociology of sports and physical education: An introductory reader* (pp. 129–147). London: Routledge Falmer.

Irlinger, P. (1979). School pupils' sport and physical activity participation and the father's socio-professional category. *Traveaux & Recherches en EPS, 5,* 113–123.

Jeziorski, R.M. (1994). *The importance of school sports in American education and socialisation.* New York, London: University Press of America

Johns, D., & Dimmock, C. (1999). The marginalization of physical education: Impoverished curriculum policy and practice in Hong Kong. *Journal of Education Policy, 14,* 363–84.

Kew, F. (1997). *Sport: Social problems and issues.* Oxford, UK: Butterworth Heinemann.

Lindner, K. J. (1995). Motivation factors in the promotion of sport participation. *Hong Kong Journal of Sports Medicine and Sports Science, 1,* 16–27.

Lindner, K. J. (1998). Sport participation by Hong Kong children and youth: Part I: Extent and nature of participation. *The Hong Kong Journal of Sports Medicine and Sports Science, 6,* 16–27.

Macfarlane, D. J. (1997). Some disturbing trends in the level of habitual physical activity in Hong Kong primary school children: Preliminary findings. *Hong Kong Journal of Sports Medicine and Sports Science, 5,* 42–46.

McManus, A. M., & Armstrong, N. (1996). Physical activity patterns of Hong Kong primary school children. *Pediatric Exercise Science, 8,* 177–178.

McPherson, B. D., Curtis, J. E., & Loy, J. W. (1989). *The social significance of sport: An introduction to the sociology of sport.* Champaign, IL: Human Kinetics.

Morris, P. (1995). *The Hong Kong school curriculum: Development, issues and policies.* Hong Kong: Hong Kong University Press.

Office of Student Affairs (1995). *A profile of new full-time undergraduate students.* Hong Kong: The University of Hong Kong.

Office of Student Affairs (1996). *A profile of new full-time undergraduate students.* Hong Kong: The University of Hong Kong.

Patriksson, G. (1981). Socialization into sport involvement. *Scandinavian Journal of Sports Science, 3,* 27–32.

Postiglione, G. A., & Lee, W. O. (Eds.) (1995). *Social change and educational development — Mainland China, Taiwan and Hong Kong.* Hong Kong: The Centre of Asian Studies of the University of Hong Kong.

Smith, M. D. (1979). Getting involved in sport: Sex differences. *International Review of the Sociology of Sport, 14,* 93–99.

Smoll, F. L., Magill, R. A., & Ash, M. J. (1988). *Children in sport* (3rd edition). Champaign, IL: Human Kinetics.

Snyder, E. E., & Spreitzer, E. (1976a). Socializing into sport: An exploratory path analysis. *Research Quarterly, 47,* 238–245.

Snyder, E. E., & Spreitzer, E. (1976b). Correlates of sport participation among adolescent girls. *Research Quarterly, 47,* 804–809.

Snyder, E. E., & Spreitzer, E. (1978). Socialization comparisons of adolescent female athletes and musicians. *Research Quarterly, 49,* 342–349.

Sofranko, A. J., & Nolan, M. F. (1972). Early life experiences and adult sport participation. *Journal of Leisure Research, 4,* 6–17.

Sohi, A. S., & Singh, K. (1986). A study of family's role as a social system in socialization of sportsmen into sports in Nigeria. In J. A. Mangan & R. B. Small (Eds.), *Sport, culture, society: International historical and sociological perspectives.* Proceedings of the VIII Commonwealth and International Conference, Glasgow.

Stroot, S.A. (2002). Socialisation and participation in sport. In A. Laker (Ed.), *The sociology of sports and physical education: An introductory reader* (pp. 129–147), London, UK: Routledge Falmer.

Weistart, J. (2001). Title IX and intercollegiate sports: equal opportunity? In

D. S. Eitzen (Ed.), *Sport in contemporary society- An anthology* (sixth edition, pp. 295–301). New York: Worth Publishers.

Wold, B., & Anderssen, N. (1992). Health promotion aspects of family and peer influences on sport participation. *International Journal of Sport Psychology, 23,* 343–359.

Wu, D. Y. H. (1996). Chinese childhood socialization. In M. H. Bond (Ed.), *The handbook of Chinese psychology* (pp. 143–154). Hong Kong: Oxford University Press.

Yamaguchi, Y. (1984). A comparative study of adolescent socialization into sport: The case of Japan and Canada. *International Review of the Sociology of Sport, 19,* 63–81.

Yang, X., Telama, R., & Laakso, L. (1996). Parents' physical activity, socio-economic status and education as predictors of physical activity and sport among children and youth. *International Review of the Sociology of Sport, 32,* 273–289.

Yoesting, D. R., & Burkhead, D. L. (1973). Significance of childhood recreation experience and adult leisure behaviour: An exploratory analysis. *Journal of Leisure Research, 5,* 25–36.

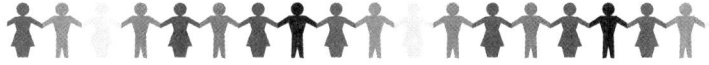

CHAPTER 10

The Influence of Policy and Practice of School Physical Education on Health-related Activity

David Johns

Introduction

The school physical education program has been identified by Sallis and McKenzie (1991) as the only institution currently responsible for promoting physical activity for all children. Because of this fact students become a target group for those who wish to identify the determining factors for physical activity. This chapter adopts the ecological model proposed by Sallis and Owen (1999) to show the diversity of forces that influence ways in which physical activity is determined. By examining the school physical education from a policy and practice perspective, it has become evident that what is planned is not what is implemented. The difficulties that physical education teachers experience become a determining factor in the low levels of activity found among Hong Kong students. This demonstrates that while schools remain the only institution responsible for promoting physical activity, they also remind us that physical activity is not determined by a single factor but by a complex set of circumstances that are beyond the control of the individual.

The influences that affect human behaviours are so complex and diverse that no single theory has so far been able to provide the depth of understanding that is required to determine what factors promote

active or sedentary lifestyles. Early psychological theories were thought
to contain the answers but they have given way to broader theories
such as the social cognitive theory of Bandura (1986). Soon after
Bandura's work had become well known, a new perspective on health
promotion programmes emerged that was referred to as an ecological
model (McLeroy, Bibeau, & Steckler,1988). The model proposed that
both individual and environmental factors should be the targets of
health promotion interventions. At the present time, the ecological
model proposed by Sallis and Owen (1999) extends these models by
providing a comprehensive framework to accommodate the variables
that are known to influence physical activity. These variables ranged
from intra-personal, community, institutional factors to public policy.
It is within this theory that this chapter has been developed to analyse
government policy and the current practice that either results from
or reacts to that policy. This will demonstrate the complex nature of
physical activity and show how diverse social structures and institutions
such as schools and governments influence its presence in the social
system. Finally, this analysis will enable more effective interventions
based on improved understanding to address the declining level of
participation in activity by young people.

Physical Education in Hong Kong

Agreement has been mounting for well over a decade that schools are
the most likely sites where behaviours leading to habitual physical
activity can be effectively developed (Boreham & Riddoch, 2001;
Haywood,1991; McGinnis, Kanner, & Degraw, 1991; Morris, 1991;
Nelson,1991; Sahota, Rudolf, Dixey, et al., 2001; Sallis & McKenzie,
1991). It is well recognized that teachers as front line workers have
access to large numbers of children who assemble regularly in an
environment that can potentially encourage and support healthy
behaviours. Children attending primary schools are particularly
impressionable because they are more responsive to behavioural
changes that are likely to continue into adolescence and beyond.
Considering that the habits of an inactive adulthood can be
possibly established during an inactive childhood, and that many
adult diseases are rooted in childhood behaviours, school physical

education can be viewed as a possible site to establish good health-related habits. Consequently, school physical education programmes have more recently been targeted for interventions, resulting in a revision of pedagogies and changes in the curriculum (Leupker, Perry, McKinley, et al. 1996; McKenzie, Sallis, Kolody, & Faucette, 1997).

Keeping in mind that schools in general have the potential to contribute to the long-term health of individuals through establishing good physical activity habits, one would expect physical education to be flourishing. Instead, the role of physical education is equivocal. This is because physical education teachers are generally very concerned about the marginality of their status (Johns & Dimmock, 1999) and even the future existence of their subject (Locke, 1998). They see themselves as structurally disadvantaged, suffering from over-commitment and burdened with administrative tasks coupled with low expectations for success (Evans & Williams, 1989; McDonald, 1999). Unfortunately, this territorial crisis, self-analysis and acquired helplessness has weakened the resolve and questioned the purpose of the profession. Paradoxically it is the curriculum planners, not the physical education teachers, who have expressed confidence in the potential of physical education to contribute to the overall develop-ment of the growing child and have included it in their plans for educational reform. Clinging to clichés about physical education, curriculum planners express their belief in physical education when they espouse objectives such as: to develop "full and individual potential in all areas covering ethics, intellect, physique, social skills and aesthetics" (Education Commission, 1999, p. 15). It is speculated that these platitudes will remain until a more effective strategy is found to implement change so that present rhetoric can be replaced by practice. At the present time this speculation does not reflect the reality, nor do existing policies translate into practice. Another paradox lies in the failed connection between ideas of policy and practices in schools and the proximity of one to the other. Such dislocation places the question of implementation in the position of becoming a determining factor of physical activity. This chapter will address the implementation problem as an example of a component of the ecology of a system in which physical activity is indirectly influenced by policies and practices.

Implementation of Change in the PE curriculum

There has been a substantial amount written about the problems of implementing the intended curriculum in the classroom (Fullan, 1998) and why policies are not implemented as planned. This has become a fertile area of analysis in a small but significant number of other Western countries because problems of curriculum implementation are remarkably similar and because the number of researchers studying the problem is relatively small (Nieto, 1998). What has emerged from these analyses are clear signs that the breakdown in the process comes at the point when teachers are given the task of transforming the technocratic planner's rhetoric into reality. The education system in Hong Kong presents a clear example of what has become a world-wide phenomenon where the gap between planning and practice has seldom been bridged.

The de-centralization of the Hong Kong education system, which for so many years was centrally controlled by a bureaucracy, has already altered the way in which the process of curriculum change takes place. In order to improve the quality of schooling, this policy of de-centralization and devolution (Dimmock & Walker, 1998), has enabled schools to assume more responsibility for their management, and allowed teachers and principals to be more actively involved in decision making (Morris, 1995). However, the direction of curriculum change emanates in documents prepared by government departments or appointed committees such as the Curriculum Development Council and not from teachers themselves. These bodies design and promote their ideas as recommendations that are eventually relayed to teachers and principals. For example, the Curriculum Development Council published a report setting out the general directions for curriculum development that include eight key learning areas of which physical education is a "fundamental concept of the major knowledge domains" (Curriculum Development Council, 2001).

While these recommendations are promising steps towards improved opportunities to ensure that school-aged youth are provided with adequate physical activity, there is little evidence that school physical education is changing. The reasons or determinants are numerous. First, the gap between policy and practice is clearly demonstrated when the agencies that set policy and write the supportive materials are working in an advisory capacity (Johns & Dimmock, 1999) and have little power or bureaucratic infrastructure to ensure the implementation of the policy or even the use of the materials. Teachers' concerns are often not about government policy and why it fails to become current practice, but about daily contingencies affecting their work. The reasons they feel no obligation to carry out the wishes of government agencies have a lot to do with the fact that there is no pressure to do so and more importantly no support to assist in the process (Barber, 1998; Fullan, 1991). Teachers have become indifferent to and cynical about the suggested curriculum and question the ability of the government to implement curriculum change. This is because government agencies lack the sensitivity regarding the will and capacity of the teachers. This applies equally to physical education teachers as it does to academic subject teachers who together represent the crucial link between policy and practice. Each teacher, regardless of their particular subject, ultimately decides what methods are to be used, the styles of learning that are employed, and most importantly, what is to be taught.

In times of change, what becomes the reality of the school curriculum is largely based on the ability of the school to resource and structure the change. Morris, Lo and Adamson (2000) have observed that the efforts towards devolution are disarticulated, promote ideological contradictions and lack an effective presentation to reveal their relevancy to the practitioner. In addition, these devolutionary and bureaucratic moves have resulted in a fragmentation of advisory policies and practices. The regular reports from the Education Commission combined with Education Department and Curriculum Development Council initiatives are supposed to create an image of coordination at the legislative, executive and bureaucratic levels of the political system. Instead, the policies are at odds and contradict one another as their proponents attempt to promote and defend one program at the expense of another (Morris et al., 2000). Consequently, the impotence of these initiatives to promote curriculum change is manifested in the way programs fade away before they have been tested, evaluated, modified and finally implemented.

Impact on physical education and active lifestyle

The implementation problems described above are not confined to Hong Kong but are shared by a global community whose interest is to make schools more effective. The discourse that Hargreaves, Leiberman, Fullan, and Hopkins (1998) have documented is an indication of the widespread interest in, as well as the complex nature of, changing policy into practice. Moreover, these difficulties of implementing curriculum change extend naturally to the challenges that face all those who are interested in promoting public health through school physical education programmes. A policy to improve health through increased activity does not mean that it can be easily translated into practice, because real change takes place only when the "beliefs, values, and ideologies held by teachers that inform their pedagogical assumptions and practices" are transformed (Sparkes, 1991, p. 2).

The problems of implementation present formidable challenges to schools that have been targeted as the most likely site to achieve the objectives of the 'health model.' Advocates of this model (Haywood, 1991; McGinnis et al., 1991; Morris, 1991; Nelson, 1991; Sallis & McKenzie, 1991) have promoted the importance and strategic relevance of school physical education and in doing so have implicitly exposed the inadequacy of existing physical education programmes. This criticism applies to programmes in many countries throughout the world including Hong Kong where the existing physical education curriculum is ill equipped to provide adequate and effective programming that would introduce students to the importance of habitual physical activity leading to more active lifestyles. Consequently, there is increasing evidence to support the concern that the population of Hong Kong is not only inactive but the habitual physical activity patterns of school age children are dramatically worse. Figure 1 reports the research by Lee (2001) on activities in the school recess that is almost identical to that reported by Johns and Ha (1999). In both studies observers recorded extremely low activity levels among the children aged 6 years to 11 years.

In the Johns and Ha (1999) study, the prevalence towards passive behaviors at home was expected, but it was found that when children

Figure 1. Recess activity patterns of Hong Kong primary school children

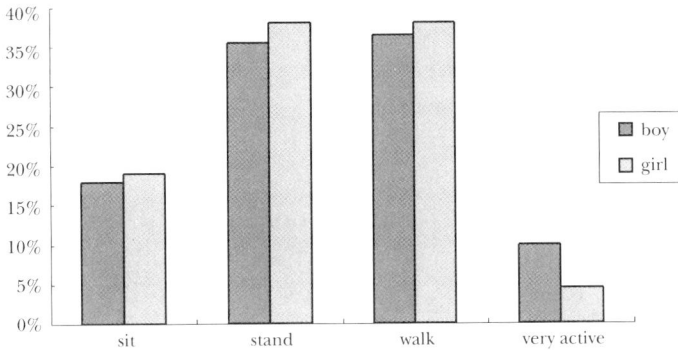

were free to play at school recess, the passive behaviours persisted as were found in Lee's study. This lack of activity is also found in the formal physical education classes. Research conducted on Hong Kong children by Macfarlane (1997), discovered that less than 4% of Hong Kong primary aged children were capable of maintaining low to medium levels of physical activity (LMPA) for 20 minutes. Furthermore, only 2% of HK primary school children were physically fit enough to achieve the modest standards recommended by Sallis and Patrick (1994) that adolescents should participate in 3–20 minutes sessions of MVPA in addition to daily lifestyle activities. Moreover, the intensity of the activities held during the required 70 minutes of physical education every 7 days in high schools seldom achieves the minimum recommended standards as only 3.4 minutes (16%) of the physical education class was devoted to vigorous activity (Macfarlane, 1997). Unfortunately, these patterns represent the lowest levels of habitual physical activity found in the literature and raises the possibility that such undesirable habitual behaviours found among primary school students will remain with them as they enter the secondary school where moderate to vigorous physical activity (MVPA) levels are seldom attained (Johns, Ha, & Macfarlane, 2001).

The results of these studies would be of no consequence if physical activity had no impact on the quality of life. However, there is compelling evidence to suggest that the burden of ill health is attributable to a lack of physical activity (Hardman, 2001) because sedentary lifestyles are closely associated with increased rates of disease. As a result, health professionals, government officials and the general public have become alarmed at the perceived health threat and subsequent medical burden posed by disorders such as obesity, diabetes, and high blood pressure.

In Hong Kong, rates of obesity in particular, match or exceed the prevalence of obesity throughout the world (Goran, 2001; World Health Organization, 1997). In addition, a recent redefinition of overweight (>23kg/m) and obese- (>26 kg/m) using the Body Mass Index (BMI) for Ethnic Chinese has increased the number of individuals who now fall in this category (World health Organization, 2000). Regardless of the standards used, rates of adult obesity that reach as high as 30–40% (Guldan et al., 1998; Leung 1995) are disturbing, because children are likely to follow similar patterns as they mature into adults. In a period of four years from 1993–1997, the percentage of obesity in boys ages 6–18 increased from 13.4% to 23% whereas girls of the same age showed a smaller percentage increase from 10.5% to 12% (Guldan, Cheung & Chui, 1998; Leung, 1995). Not only is obesity difficult to cure in adults, there is mounting evidence to suggest that it is strongly linked to high blood pressure and cardiovascular diseases in Hong Kong Chinese (Lee, Critchley, Chan, et al., 2000; Thomas, Critchley, Tomlinson, et al., 2000). In addition, the prevalence of type-2 diabetes in Hong Kong has increased sharply from 7.7% to 8.9% between 1990 and 1995 (Cockram, 2000).

The rising rates and early onset of diseases such as obesity and type-2 diabetes (developed before 30 years of age) are the results of sudden and widespread changes in the lifestyle of Hong Kong population. They also reflect the warnings that have already been given by a wide range of researchers who are consistent in their appeal to the schools to assist in preventing further deterioration in the general health of children. For example, in 1987, the Committee on Sport Medicine and the Committee of School Health of the American Academy of Pediatrics recommended to pediatricians to appeal to local school boards to maintain and if possible, increase the physical fitness component of school physical education programmes (Nelson, 1991). The warnings have continued since that time but there is little evidence to suggest that much progress has been made. In Hong Kong school physical education has remained a marginalized school subject that is sometimes replaced by more academic courses especially around the time when examination preparation is deemed to take precedence. When it is permitted to function as a school subject, the duration for primary schools only amounts two 35 minute classes. Considering that large proportions of the class time are spent on organisational and managerial tasks (Macfarlane, 1997) the time spent actively engaged in physical activity is negligible in terms of its contribution to health. In secondary schools a single period of 75 minutes is provided and that is supposed to occur once in every 7-day school cycle of which there are 21 for the school year. A 7-day cycle not only denies students the opportunity to participate in a weekly class but invariably, with school examinations and public holidays, it reduces their participation to less than two periods per month. In some schools, senior students may receive as little as 6 physical education classes per year. While schools claim that they offer physical education to all students, such an arrangement would not provide enough regular physical activity to have any positive effect on their health.

The Ideal Physical Education Curriculum

The school physical education program has been identified by Sallis and McKenzie as "the only institution currently responsible for promoting physical activity for all children" (1991, p. 127). It is considered to be the most ideally structured programme in modern societies in which it is possible to train children to function effectively as adults. However, when we focus on school physical education as a site for change to improve the level and intensity of exercise, there is considerable debate. The discourse over what should be taught in physical education has not only broadened with the introduction of new curricula (Curtner-Smith, 1999) but has served as a platform to justify and protect existing roles for physical education (Haywood, 1991; McGinnis et al.,1991; Morris, 1991; Nelson,1991; Sallis & McKenzie, 1991; Tinning, 2001). Nevertheless, there is agreement among physical educators that a health–related physical education programme is desirable, and children should not be denied the opportunity to participate. Sallis and McKenzie (1991) suggested that physical educators should adopt a new role and pursue a goal that reflects current public health concerns and ways to encourage lifetime of physical activity. However, teachers vary in what they believe is the most important objective for physical education. Some believe in physical fitness, others suggest motor skill development, and some feel that the enhancement of self-esteem is not merely an outcome but an important benefit of participation. Difficulties also arise if exercises suitable for adults are applied to primary school age children. Very little research has been conducted on this specific age group and therefore the application of adult principles of fitness lack the evidence to endorse their safety or effectiveness for children. Other difficulties have been raised concerning the primary school physical education curriculum that has traditionally included dance and games. Some argue that physical education can provide aerobic benefits through exercise and games but instructional experience is also essential before active participation can be expected. Obviously a balance must be achieved between teaching children skills that are essential to participation and maintain a high level of moderate to vigorous activity. To motivate young people and to develop an active lifestyle that will continue into adulthood requires a developmental approach. By means of "age/ability appropriate and sequential lessons" (Haywood, 1991, p. 155), primary and secondary schools students are provided with a knowledge base about exercise and health in which every year is sequentially linked in order that health-related primary school programmes will ultimately link up with healthy adult lifestyles. To instill the desire to be active requires a greater understanding of what motivates individuals to select one lifestyle over another. Forcing students into a physical fitness regime is not the answer.

Summary

In this chapter there has been an attempt to demonstrate that it is unlikely that a single influence can determine the level and frequency of human physical activity. There is an assertion that the factors that facilitate or prevent such behaviours are complex and cannot be reduced to simplistic explanations. It is more likely that the low level of physical activity found among youth in Hong Kong is due to a combination of social, cultural and environmental forces. These forces can be divided into those that are consistent with the consensus statements about physical activity that have been reached by a wide range of observers (Sallis & Owen, 1999) and those that are specific to the Chinese culture. For example, the lack of physical space can be considered a universal barrier that most likely impacts on all youth regardless of their location or cultural beliefs, whereas the Confucian ethic that runs deep in the way Chinese children are brought up may have a profound but unique effect on physical activity patterns of youth in this region of China. This specific influence will be discussed in Chapter 11.

Identifying the possible effects of physical, cultural and social barriers on these behaviours is a useful step forward but fails to transform patterns of behaviour. What is required is further analysis and identification of ways to modify behaviour taking into consideration that some barriers cannot be dismantled while others are potentially removable. Therefore, the need to understand the difference between what can and what cannot be changed is essential before interventions can be designed that aim at increasing activity as a lifestyle change. Because schools exist to change young people, it is more likely that their behaviours can be altered substantially and permanently than it is to focus on trying to change the minds of school authorities, architects and governments regarding the construction of ideal facilities. In other words, it is more productive to focus on changing social structures and institutions rather than the physical environments in which they exist. The school physical education programme is a socially constructed institution and therefore should be flexible enough to be changed in ways that profoundly affect the habitual behaviours of young people.

While the focus of the school physical education discourse is often fractured, the institution of schooling continues to be the most likely site where change can be substantial and lasting to affect future generations. Schools have the potential to determine the role of physical activity in the lives of children, and public health workers justifiably are calling for the necessary changes to realize this goal. However, such a goal can only be realized if government departments of education are willing to adopt policies that can be transformed into classroom reality. At the present time, an active lifestyle remains an unachieved goal for many individuals whose lives are bombarded with alternatives that tend to exacerbate the inactivity problem rather than reduce it. In Hong Kong children are nurtured in an extreme urban environment that places great emphasis on materialism, consumerism and less on life quality, well-being and health. Until we can raise the consciousness of individuals to be discriminating in their choice of lifestyle, other cultural imperatives and social preferences will continue to overshadow the significance of health-related behaviours that impact on the individual's health status especially the generation that is currently of school age.

References

Bandura, A. (1986). *Social foundations of thought and action: A social cognitive theory.* Englewood Cliffs, NJ: Prentice-Hall.

Barber, M. (1998). National strategies for educational reform: Lessons from the British experience since 1988. In A. Hargreaves, A. Leiberman, M. Fullan, & D. Hopkins (Eds.), *International handbook of educational change* (pp. 743–767). London, UK: Kluwer Academic Publishers.

Boreham, C., & Riddoch, C. (2001). The physical activity, fitness and health of children. *Journal of Sport Sciences, 19,* 915–929.

Cockram C. (2000). The epidemiology of diabetes mellitus in theAsia-Pacific region. *Hong Kong Medicine Journal, 6,* 43–52.

Curriculum Development Council (2001). *Learning to learn: Lifelong learning and whole-person development.* Hong Kong: Author.

Curtner-Smith, M. D. (1999). The more things change the more they stay the same: Factors influencing teachers' interpretations and delivery of national curriculum physical education. *Sport, Education and Society, 4,* 75–97.

Dimmock, C., & Walker, A. (1998). Transforming Hong Kong schools: Trends and emerging issues. *Journal of Educational Administration, 36,* 476–508.

Education Commission (1997, September). *Report No. 7. (ECR7). Quality school education.* Hong Kong: The Government Printer.

Education Commission (1999). *Education blueprint for the 21st century.* Hong Kong: The Government Printer.

Evans, J., & Williams, T. (1989). Moving up and getting out: The classed, gendered career opportunities of physical education teachers. In

T. Templin & P. Schempp (Eds.), *Socialization in physical education: Learning to teach* (pp. 235–249). Indianapolis, IN: Benchmark Press.

Fullan, M. (1991). *The new meaning of educational change.* London: Cassell.

Fullan, M. (1998). *The meaning of education change: A quarter of a century of learning.* In A. Hargreaves, A. Leiberman, M. Fullan, & D. Hopkins (Eds), *International handbook of educational change* (pp. 214–228). London: Kluwer Academic Publishers.

Goran, M. (2001). Metabolic precursors and effects of obesity in children: A decade of progress, 1990–1999. *American Journal of Clinical Nutrition, 73,* 158–171.

Guldan, G. S., Cheung, I. L. T., & Chui, K. K. H. (1998). Childhood obesity in Hong Kong: Embracing an unhealthy lifestyle before puberty. *International Journal of Obesity, 22*(Supplement), S49.

Hargreaves, A., Leiberman, A., Fullan, M., & Hopkins, D. (Eds.) (1998). *International handbook of educational change.* London: Kluwer Academic Publishers.

Haywood, K. (1991). The role of physical education in the development of active lifestyles. *Research Quarterly for Exercise and Sport, 62,* 151–156.

Johns, D., & Dimmock, C. (1999). The marginalization of physical education: Impoverished curriculum policy and practice in Hong Kong. *Journal of Education Policy, 14,* 363–84.

Johns, D. P., & Ha, A. (1999). Home and recess physical activity of Hong Kong children. *Research Quarterly of Exercise and Sport, 70,* 319–323.

Johns, D., Ha, A. S. C., & Macfarlane, D. (2001). Raising activity levels: A multi-dimensional analysis of curriculum change. *Sport, Education & Society, 6,* 199–210.

Lee, K. H. F. (2001) *An analysis of school playground behaviors in Hong Kong primary school children.* Unpublished M. Phil. dissertation, The Chinese University of Hong Kong.

Lee, Z. S., Critchley, J. A., Chan, N., Chan, J. C., Anderson, P. J., Thomas, G. N., Ko, G. T., Young, R. P., Chan, T. Y., Cockram, C. S., & Tomlinson, B. (2000). Obesity is the key determinant of cardiovascular risk factors in the Hong Kong Chinese population: Cross sectional clinic-based study. *Hong Kong Medical Journal, 6,* 13–23.

Leung, S. S. (1995). Childhood obesity in Hong Kong. *Hong Kong Journal of Paediatrics, 1*(supplement), 63–68.

Leupker, R. V., Perry, C. L., McKinley, S. M., Nader, P. R., Parcel, G. S., Stone,

E. J., Webber, L. S., Elder, J. P., Feldman, H. A., Johnson, C.C., Kelder, S. H., & Wu, M. (1996). Outcomes of a field trial to improve children's dietary patterns and physical activity. The child and adolescent trial for cardiovascular health (CATCH). *Journal of American Medical Association*, 275, 768–776.

Lindner, K. J. (1997). Sport participation in Hong Kong children and youth: Rates and reasons. *Hong Kong: Hong Kong Sport Development Board*.

Locke, L. (1998). Advice, stories and myths: The reactions of a cliff jumper. *Quest, 50*, 238–48.

Macdonald, D. (1999). The "professional" work of experienced physical education teachers. *Research Quarterly for Exercise and Sport, 70*, 41–54.

Macfarlane, D. J. (1997). Some disturbing trends in the levels of habitual physical activity in Hong Kong primary school children: Preliminary findings. *Hong Kong Journal of Sports Medicine & Sports Science, 5*, 42–46.

McGinnis, J. M., Kanner, L., & Degraw, C. (1991). Physical educator's role in achieving national health objectives. *Research Quarterly for Exercise and Sport, 62*, 138-142.

McLeroy, K., Bibeau, D., Steckler, A. (1988). An ecological perspective on health promotion programs. Health Education Quarterly, 15(4), 351–177.

McKenzie, T. L., Sallis, J. F., Kolody, B., & Faucette, F. N. (1997). Long-term effects of a physical education curriculum and staff development program: SPARK. *Research Quarterly for Sport and Exercise, 68*, 280–291.

Morris, H. (1991). The role of physical education in public health. *Research Quarterly for Exercise and Sport, 62*, 143–147.

Morris, P. (1995). *The Hong Kong school curriculum: Development, issues and policies*. Hong Kong: Hong Kong University Press.

Morris, P., Lo, M. L., & Adamson, B. (2000). Improving schools in Hong Kong. In B. Adamson, T. Kwan, & K. K. Chan (Eds.), *Changing the curriculum: The impact of reform on primary schooling in Hong Kong* (pp. 245–262). Hong Kong: Hong Kong University Press.

Nelson, M. (1991). The role of physical education and children's activity in public health. *Research Quarterly for Exercise and Sport, 62*, 148–150.

Nieto, S. (1998). Cultural difference and educational change in a sociopolitical context'. In A. Hargreaves, A. Leiberman, M. Fullan, & D. Hopkins (Eds.), *International handbook of educational change* (pp. 418–439). London: Kluwer Academic Publishers.

Sahota, S. P., Rudolf, M., Dixey, R., Hill, A., Barth, J., & Cade J. (2001).

Randomised control trial of primary school based intervention to reduce risk factors for obesity. *British Medical Journal, 323,* 1–5.

Sallis, J. F., & McKenzie, T. L. (1991). Physical educator's role in public health. *Research Quarterly for Exercise and Sport, 62,* 124–37.

Sallis, J., & Patrick, K. (1994). Physical activity guidelines for adolescents: Consensus statement. *Pediatric Exercise Science, 6,* 302–314.

Sallis , J., & Owen, N. (1999). *Physical activity and behavioural medicine.* London: Sage.

Sparkes, A. (1991). Curriculum change: On gaining a sense of perspective. In N. Armstrong & A. Sparkes (Eds.). *Issues in physical education* (pp. 1–19). London: Cassell.

Thomas, G., Critchley, J., Tomlinson, B., Anderson, P., Lee, Z., & Chan, J. (2000). Obesity, independent of insulin resistance, is a major determinant of blood pressure in normoglycemic Hong Kong Chinese. *Metabolism, 49,* 1523–1528.

Tinning, R. (2001, June). *Physical education and the making of citizens: Considering the pedagogical work of physical education in contemporary times.* JoséMarié Cagigal Lecture, AIESEP International Congress, Taipei, Taiwan.

World Health Organization (1997). *Preventing and managing the global epidemic.* Geneva: Author

World Health Organization. (2000). The Asia-Pacific Perspective:

Re-defining Obesity and Its Treatment. WHO: Health Communications Australia PtyLimited.

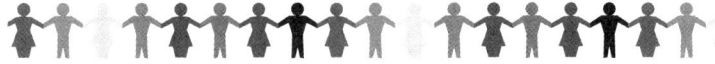

CHAPTER 11

The Influence of Physical, Cultural and Social Environments on Health-related Activity

David Johns and Patricia Vertinsky

Introduction

This chapter focuses upon how health-related physical activity may be influenced by psychological, cultural and social factors which also interact with the physical environment. In keeping with the ecological model suggested by Sallis and Owen, (1999), we adopt the perspective that intuitively considers these influences to have a significant bearing on the habits of individuals in their daily lives. While it is impossible to consider all factors that are likely to shape the type and amount of physical activity in which individuals participate, it is useful to examine influences that are likely to be taken for granted and therefore overlooked. These influences are different from those described in Chapter 10, where school reform policy, designed to improve school effectiveness and the quality of physical education, fails to do so in practice. In this chapter we look primarily at cultural and social forces that go unnoticed, or are generally accepted without question in everyday life, in order to illustrate how beliefs and values act and are acted upon within the social, cultural and physical environment.

We will first examine the physical environment to show that although severe physical limitations shape the ways in which social life in Hong Kong is structured, cultural and social values also influence the ways in which the physical environment is utilized. Our attention will then turn to the interactions in family life to illustrate how strong cultural values shape widely held beliefs about the nurture and education of children. Although these beliefs are based on ancient teachings that can be traced back to Confucian times (and are no longer explicitly identified as such in everyday life), they are detectable to the careful observer. In our effort to explain how these factors influence the relatively low level of physical activity reported in this book, we will show how individuals interpret cultural and social values within the ecology of the urban setting of Hong Kong.

The Physical Environment

The ecological model used to study the factors affecting our health considers the constellation of lifestyle behaviours as a multidimensional influence that constrains behaviour through either facilitation or prevention. The model includes the consideration of the physical environment that, according to Humpel, Owen and Leslie (2000), is "among the least understood of the known influences on physical activity" (p. 188). The physical environment of Hong Kong is a particularly striking example of a dense urban development that has a significant impact on human behaviour, especially health-related physical activity. From the urban designer's point of view, the effectiveness of the transportation and accommodation of 7 million people in their everyday lives is nothing short of miraculous. However, this miracle of human ingenuity to house and move people has resulted in the significant reduction of the need to walk because of the various forms of transportation as describe by Macfarlane in Chapter 5. Individuals travel rapidly from home to work, shops and restaurants on trains, buses, ferries and taxis that are located in such a way that the need to walk has been greatly reduced or eliminated altogether. The logistics of speed detach the body from the spaces through which it moves, and pacify it physically (Sennett, 1994). Consequently, physical activity in the form of purposeful, vigorous walking is reduced to a minimum.

No studies that we know of have been conducted specifically on the effect that the built environment of Hong Kong has on physical activity. However, if the ecological model is applied to the setting of

Hong Kong, one can see that several influences may be operating. One obvious influence is the accessibility of facilities that would perhaps encourage individuals to avail themselves of the opportunity to become more active if more space (and more appropriate space) was available for people to participate in a safe environment. This is the case in some of the housing developments where older citizens can be seen practicing various forms of Tai Chi in the early morning, and both Hong Kong Island and the New Territories boast extensive hiking paths available for hikers with the means, the access and the interest. Of course access to green space involves much more than physical availability; there are significant economic, social and cultural factors, which help explain why different social groups seek out or are able to use and enjoy the rural surroundings of Hong Kong's urban centers regardless of climatic issues.

Within the urban areas, many of the modern housing estates have included swimming pools and formal playgrounds with installed fixed play equipment. However, these examples cannot be considered the norm, particularly in the older estates in Hong Kong where outdoor facilities are inadequate or poorly maintained. It is only in the more affluent parts of the city that thought and care has been taken to develop facilities that encourage outdoor activity. Safety is also a concern expressed by parents who are reluctant to send their children out to play in unprotected areas where they may encounter undesirable influences. Thus landscapes which may appear highly conducive to play and sports become, for some, landscapes of fear and anxiety. Women are often fearful to venture into unprotected areas for fear of harassment or other dangers, and fear of injury is a further deterrent to parents of children playing in playgrounds or on the street. All too often the shopping malls become the arena of choice for adolescents and families who can spend their free time strolling, shopping, socializing and eating in air-conditioned enclosures full of other people.

School Facilities

As we have seen in the previous chapter, schools are now considered to be a major institution where children can be introduced to and are able to maintain a programme of physical activity. Unfortunately, Hong Kong faces some unique and almost insurmountable problems with regard to the built environment and education. Unlike many North American and European settings, Hong Kong's communities are located on some of the most expensive real estate in the world, and exist in some of the most densely populated urban environments to be found (Johns & Dimmock, 1999). The demand on land use is extraordinarily high as demonstrated in the allocation of land for schools. Typically, schools are allocated between 6200m^2 and 6950m^2 of space, and in the case of primary schools they have to be located within 0.4km measured radially from residential areas (Hong Kong Government Planning Standards, 1998). This restriction of area represents between 5 and 20 times less space for schools than that demanded by many school boards in the United States (Bucher & Krotee, 1998). Limited space therefore is a major constraint upon facilities for physical activity, predisposing youngsters to constrain their own bodily movements, for, as Bourdieu (1984, p. 474) points out, "one's relationship to the social world and one's proper place in it is expressed in the space one is able to claim with one's body in physical space". Dance teachers in Hong Kong have noticed this, when given freedom to explore space in the dance studio, students often flock together rather than seeking out an open space.

Typically, school playgrounds are located between tall buildings and are used by the public who may wander across the playground in the middle of a PE lesson. Teachers in these schools are often frustrated by the lack of facilities and their location, as reported below (personal communication):

Our main problem is facilities; we just don't have enough court space or open space to conduct our programmes. And even if we had, we have to be careful in the playground because someone may throw an object from a window on the 23rd floor of a surrounding apartment block. And as if that is not dangerous enough, then we have to stop classes when the pollution rating is too high, because the students could get breathing problems.

Schools usually have one or two play areas that have painted lines for school sports such as basketball, volleyball and badminton. Even when outdoor activity spaces are provided they are limited and there is little or no protection from the elements. In some schools improvements have been made to the playground surfaces by replacing concrete with all-weather surfaces but during the wet seasons even these areas become unusable. The mean yearly temperature and relative humidity of 23C and 77% respectively ensures that strenuous outdoor activity will be uncomfortably hot and result in profuse sweating. With few schools providing showers and adequate hygiene and changing facilities, it is not surprising that young people are reluctant to participate in vigorous physical education. Moreover, high UV ratings combined with a reluctance to be exposed to the sun and darken the skin form other reasons why many avoid outdoor activity where possible. In addition, air quality is frequently affected by pollution caused by vehicle emissions that reach levels that provoke public warnings not to exercise out of doors. When pollution levels are extreme, physical education classes are suspended because there are no purpose-built, climate controlled gymnasiums that could provide safe and comfortable conditions for students to participate without suffering heat stroke or respiratory problems.

Even when the outdoor playgrounds are useable, there are tight controls over school playgrounds, particularly in primary schools. Yi-Fu Tuan (1979, p. 99) has said that "a successfully designed playground is one in which children are conscious only of their own kinaesthetic joy and the potential field for action." Institutionally, notes Thomson (2004), in her study of children's school playgrounds in England, the playground space supposedly represents an area set aside for childish activities, implying an engagement with children and their needs and habits. Ideally it is an area independent of the classroom where children can express themselves more freely than in other places in the school — a place for play and physicality, not work. In reality, the space of the playground is more often used as a 'technique of power, ' to control and monitor children's bodies. Foucault (1977) has illuminated how this takes place in institutions such as schools through taken-for-granted practices in which bodies are disciplined and rendered docile. In this sense the playground often becomes simply an exchange of one educational surrounding for another — a place of spatial discipline to monitor and train children's behaviour. This is what Lee (2001) found in her study of Hong Kong school playgrounds. She discovered that the principal, in the schools she observed, required staff and student helpers to police the playground to ensure that no boisterous activities took place. Her observations revealed that students spent the recess period engaged in eating and at best walking slowly around the playground. In another study, Johns and Ha (1999) found that the lack of physical activity was combined with a series of social reinforcers that encouraged students to be inactive and to use recess time to eat snacks purchased in the school tuck shop. Even activities not requiring large areas of playground space such as the use of balls, skipping ropes or other harmless articles were discouraged or absent from the playground.

Taken together, these limitations demonstrate the zeal with which many Hong Kong educators employ restrictive rules and forms of surveillance that promote quiet areas, demand frequent lining up, and effectively restrict the natural movement of children in the name of safety and control. In most of the 12 schools observed by Lee, teachers, instructed by the school principal, feared the consequences of allowing children to run or move naturally, and as a measure to reduce this risk eliminated all movement beyond walking. The tight control also reflects the willingness of teachers (or demands placed upon them) to restrict rather than find ways to facilitate activity and their fears of litigation and parental complaints. This is consistent with the low value that is placed on physical activity and the limited role that it is allowed to play in the natural development of children. The lack of response in the design of buildings and the provision of facilities also demonstrates how policy is shaped by a set of values that views physical activity as not deserving of facilities that in many Western countries are considered to be a necessity. To be fair, physical education is not the only subject with a facility that is not provided. Up until recently, many other school subjects involving information technology, science laboratories, music and art were also poorly resourced. Nevertheless, the absence of facilities and equipment is normal in schools with respect to physical education and reflects a public policy that marginalizes physical activity as an unnecessary and unimportant activity for young people.

Culturally based determinants

In *Spaces of Hope* (2000) David Harvey points out that, as we collectively produce our cities, so we collectively produce ourselves. Projects concerning what we want our cities (and the spaces within it) to become are, therefore, projects about who we want to become. Thus built space is not just a container of bodies and identities but is a constitutive element in them. The actual materiality of bodies (and the desire and ability to participate in physical activity) is constructed and inscribed by the environment. Urban spaces take form largely from the ways people experience their own bodies. (Sennett, 1994). In this sense we can understand the built environment as one which reflects the received wisdom of clients, sponsors and consumers about class divisions, gender roles, and desired social practices and embodied experiences. From this perspective we can now turn to an examination of cultural values and psychological traits that illustrate how the severe physical limitations in Hong Kong are but one of many influences that affect physical activity. Ecological influences that are likely to affect the physical behaviours of individuals are more psychologically/ culturally bound to the beliefs and values that are deeply embedded in the individual's psyche. The origins of these beliefs are to be found in the ancient teachings of Confucian scholars who first wrote "in plain language to guide parents in providing their children with proper discipline and educational instruction at home" (Wu, 1996, p. 144). Compared to modern standards and practices, early Chinese training focused on self-control and discipline particularly in those families of the 'gentry' class (Wu, 1996). Emphasis was placed on deportment and proper demeanor, to restrain the body and demonstrate reverence in the presence of adults. The outward appearance and the training of the physical were restrictive in that physical activities and boisterous actions such as "leaping, arguing, joking, slouching, or using vulgar language" (Dardness, 1991, p. 79) were discouraged. These attitudes towards the moderation of what today would be considered normal behaviours for exuberant youth, have somehow been 'bred in the bone' and continue to be manifested in the way young females and to a lesser extent males deport themselves even though they are no longer formally taught. This is particularly obvious in the way female students in physical education classes move with constraint when playing games such as volleyball and basketball. Although there is a pronounced control exhibited among adolescent females when they engage in physical activity this is less obvious among adolescent males who assume an approach to physical activity that would typify a Western physical education class. This has been observed by the male and female physical education teachers that we have talked with, who report frustration with the apparent lack of enthusiasm that female students in particular show for any kind of physical activity.

The reasons for this are complex. When we look at the historical development of school physical education in Hong Kong, one can readily see its colonial heritage and its gendered contours. It is well established in the West, from where Hong Kong curriculum models were imported, that physical education plays a critical role in the development of masculinity and femininity. Indeed it is a prime site for the social and cultural construction of gender (Dewar, 1987). Perceived physical differences and abilities between boys and girls have traditionally formed the bedrock upon which school physical education programs have been designed and implemented (Vertinsky, 1992). This is readily apparent in Hong Kong secondary schools where physical education is largely a sex-segregated affair providing a context in which gendered identities and separate gendered cultures develop and come to appear natural. Although popular perception has it that equality between men and women, girls and boys in Hong Kong has been more or less achieved, gender continues to remain a basis of segregation, evaluation and resource distribution in the schools as elsewhere in society (Cheung, 1997). Sex stereotyping of sport activities constrain learning and interest and the low motivation and participation of girls in health enhancing physical activity has become an area of pressing concerns. Hong Kong society, despite its modern outlook is permeated with traditionalism where women's roles are defined by traditional Chinese values and the family plays an important role in supporting the traditional images of woman as the weaker and subordinate sex. Most of the girls in secondary schools, says Lo (1996), accept their gender definition as quiet, soft, physically inferior and non-athletic. They act as true defenders of the feminine values of tenderness, nurture and compassion that probably were generated from their family. How far physical education teachers are sensitized to these stereotyping concepts and discriminatory practices or to an understanding of the construction of the curriculum they implement (and thus the reproduction of gendered bodies) is a matter of conjecture.

Where younger children are concerned, traditional Chinese early training methods have given way to new rearing practices in which children are 'drowned with love' and, according to some critics, parents allow their "affection for their children to interfere with their disciplinary responsibilities" (Wu, 1996, p. 147). The prevalence of maids and grandparents taking care of young children further exacerbates the level of control over the child's physicality. Maids, dictated to by mothers and grandparents are under severe constraints to keep children happy and safe, catering to their wishes, overdressing them and not infrequently carrying them around, even at kindergarten age (Salaff, 1995). When the child is old enough to attend formal schooling, the relationship between parent and child shifts from parental over-indulgence (Stevenson & Lee, 1996) to one that (although in decline) is strongly influenced by filial piety, an ethic that "surpasses all other ethics" in terms of its historical continuity and the encompassing and imperative nature of its precepts (Ho, 1996, p. 155). Filial piety plays an important "instrumental role in shaping personality, social behaviour and socio-political institutions" (Ho, 1996, p. 156) and as a consequence, has a profound influence over the child's school-related academic and physical performances.

The relationship between filial piety and education is further influenced by a neo-Confucian ethic (Vogel, 1991) that places great emphasis on academic achievement by means of diligence, hard work, and effort. The Confucian ethic elevated scholarship above all other stations in traditional Chinese life especially those that were associated with farmers, merchants and labourers (Stevenson & Lee, 1996). It seems that these traditional values have not faded from the Chinese psyche although the forms in which they are manifested may have changed. In the modern urban family in Hong Kong, the effect of filial piety combined with the Confucian emphasis on scholarship is pronounced. Even today, children are willing to devote large amounts of time to academic pursuits, placing their own preferences behind the wishes of their parents in order to do well in school. Of course, while dutiful devotion to study often results in good academic outcomes that please parents, such piety often impacts negatively on physical activity which is considered to be a distraction and a time waster. While there is no evidence to suggest that engaging in regular sports programmes has any detrimental effects on academic performance (Lindner, 1999) [indeed, physical educators have historically claimed that physical training enhances academic performance, following a tradition that goes back to the Greeks], Hong Kong parents in general continue to be confused over the impact that participation in sport may have on academic performance. It seems that there is a general notion among many parents and teachers that a young person cannot engage and excel in both areas of endeavour, and to be a student/athlete is regarded as an unlikely combination. Moreover, it has been shown that participation in sport and physical activities drops as the level of schooling rises (Lindner, 1999), thus further determining the patterns of inactivity. Sport involvement and health benefits that accompany such participation are sacrificed in case they would interfere with academic progress.

Apart from the belief that the young are unlikely to succeed academically if they engage in sports, the act of participating in physical activity is also considered to be antithetical to cognitive development and certainly inferior to endeavours of the mind. According to Johns and Dimmock (1999) physical education remains a marginalized school subject because it is associated with physical hard work and resembles the labour endured by social classes who were not scholars. Naturally, physical education is regarded as less important than core academic subjects such as mathematics, science and language that are accorded more timetable allocation at the expense of cultural subjects like physical education (Morris, 1998). Class and family alliance have played a very important role in shaping bodily practices such as sport and physical recreation, often trumping gender issues in its importance. For example, Dong (2003) points out that in China women's and girls' involvement in sport has been seen less as an intrusion into the male preserve and a threat to their sexuality than a class transgression. What matters is the importance placed by traditional Confucian values on women's reproductive ability, making their bodies special objects of knowledge and surveillance. Confucian gender values tend to assume that the normative female body is fertile and that reproductive problems are the fault of the woman and her actions (and lifestyle) (Brownwell, 1995). Thus infertility is highly stigmatizing and women and girls learn to be very cautious in indulging in bodily practices such as sport and vigorous physical activity that they perceive might damage their reproductive health. At the level of the classroom, or gymnasium, or swimming pool, these anxieties are manifested in the girls' desire to avoid physical activity during menstruation (Handwerker, 1995).

These structural and ideological issues associated with the school curriculum are major factors that influence the intensity, frequency and irregular patterns of physical activity, and are most likely to be associated with the low levels of physical activity that have been noted by several researchers (Johns & Ha, 1999; Macfarlane, 1997). Because physical inactivity is now recognized as a major risk factor for cardiovascular disease (Hardman, 2001), it would seem logical to place a greater emphasis on physical education programmes to bring about behavioural changes. Although "the question of whether physical activity or fitness is most strongly related to health status remains unresolved" (Boreham & Riddoch, 2001, p. 916), the shift from fitness and health to health-related physical activity seems a reasonable approach to take. Attempting to establish an ethos rather than an edict that encourages a physically active lifestyle seems much more likely to succeed in the reduction of sedentary lives that may well follow today's children into adulthood. However, the health message, which has been delivered to secondary schools via battery fitness testing has been shown to be less than successful to date in promoting the advantages of physical activity, especially for girls. Furthermore, despite the stated focus upon health and fitness, the content and mechanisms of physical education remain largely concerned with sport and, increasingly now that Hong Kong has become a special administrative region of China, the use of school programmes as a nursery for fostering elite sports talent rather than sport for all. Clearly then it is not simply the physical environment that inhibits physical activity. Rather it is how the ecological balance of individuals living within the dense urban environment of postmodern Hong Kong is reached and maintained that is also a powerful determinant of modes of embodiment such as health-related physical activity.

References

Boreham, C., & Riddoch, C. (2001). The physical activity, fitness and health of children. *Journal of Sport Sciences, 19*, 915–929.

Bourdieu, P. (1984). *Distinction. A social critique of the judgement of taste.* Cambridge, MA: Harvard University Press.

Brownwell, S. (1995). *Training the body for China: Sports in the moral order of the People's Republic.* Chicago, IL: University of Chicago Press.

Bucher, C. A., & Krotee, M. L. (1998). *Management of physical education and sport.* New York, NY: WCB/Mcgraw-Hill.

Cheung, F. (Ed.) (1997). *Engendering Hong Kong society.* Hong Kong: The Chinese University Press.

Dewar, A. (1987). The social construction of gender in physical education. *Women's Studies International Forum, 10*, 453–465.

Dong, J. (2003). *Women and sport in modern China.* London: Frank Cass.

Foucault, M. (1977). *Discipline and punish: The birth of the prison.* London: Allen Lane.

Handwerker, L. (1995). The hen that can't lay an egg: Conceptions of female infertility in China. In J. Terry & J. Urla (Eds.). *Deviant bodies: Critical perspectives on difference in science and popular culture* (pp. 358–386). Bloomington, IN: Indiana University Press.

Hardman, A. E. (2001). Physical activity and health: current issues and research needs. *International Journal of Epidemiology, 30*, 1193–1197.

Harvey, D. (2000). *Spaces of hope.* Berkeley, CA: University of California Press.

Ho, D. Y. F. (1986). Chinese patterns of socialization. In M. H. Bond (Ed.), *The psychology of the Chinese people.* Hong Kong: Oxford University Press.

Hong Kong Government Planning Standards (1998). *Hong Kong planning standards and guidelines.* Hong Kong: The Government Press.

Humpel, N., Owen, N., & Leslie, E. (2000). Environmental factors associated with adults' participation in physical activity. *American Journal of Preventive Medicine, 22*, 188–199.

Johns, D., & Dimmock, C. (1999). The marginalization of physical education: Impoverished curriculum policy and practice in Hong Kong. *Journal of Education Policy, 14*, 363–84.

Johns, D. P., & Ha, A. (1999). Home and recess physical activity of Hong Kong children. *Research Quarterly of Exercise and Sport, 70*, 319–323.

Lee, K. H. F. (2001) *An analysis of school playground behaviors in Hong Kong primary school children.* Unpublished M. Phil. Dissertation, The Chinese University of Hong Kong.

Lindner, K. J. (1997). Sport participation in Hong Kong children and youth: Rates and reasons. *Hong Kong: Hong Kong Sport Development Board.*

Lindner, K. J. (1999). Sport participation and perceived academic performance of school children and youth. *Pediatric Exercise Science, 10*, 129–143.

Lindner, K. J. (2002). The activity participation - academic performance relationship revisited: Perceived and actual performance, and the effect of banding (academic tracking). *Pediatric Exercise Science, 14*, 155–169.

Lo, H. Y. S. (1996). The effects of gender role stereotypes on the choice of sport of secondary school girls in Hong Kong. In D. J. Macfarlane (Ed.), *Gender issues in sport and exercise* (p. 88). Hong Kong: The University of Hong Kong.

Macfarlane, D. J. (1997). Some disturbing trends in the levels of habitual physical activity in Hong Kong primary school children: Preliminary findings. *Hong Kong Journal of Sports Medicine & Sports Science, 5*, 42–46.

Morris, P. (1998). School knowledge, the state and the market: An analysis of the Hong Kong secondary school curriculum. In P. Stimpson & P. Morris (Eds.), *Curriculum and assessment for Hong Kong: Two components, one system* (pp. 141–170). Hong Kong: Open University of Hong Kong Press.

Salaff, J. (1995). *Working daughters of Hong Kong: Filial piety or power in the family.* New York, NY: Columbia University Press.

Sallis, J., & Owen, N. (1999). *Physical activity & behavioral medicine.* London: Sage.

Sennett, R. (1994). *Flesh and stone. The body and the city in western civilization.* New York, NY: W. W. Norton.

Stevenson, H. W., & Lee, S-Y. (1996). The academic achievement of Chinese students. In M. H. Bond (Ed.), *The handbook of Chinese psychology* (pp. 124–142). Hong Kong: Oxford University Press.

Thomson, S. (2004). Just another classroom: Observations of primary school playgrounds. In P. Vertinsky & J. Bale (Eds.), *Sites of sport: Space, place and experience* . London: Frank Cass.

Tuan, Y-F. (1979). Thought and landscape: The eye and the mind. In D. W.

Meining (Ed.), *The interpretation of ordinary landscapes* (p. 99). New York, NY: Oxford University Press.

Vertinsky, P. (1992). Reclaiming space, revisioning the body: The quest for gender sensitive physical education. *Quest, 44,* 373–396.

Vogel, E. (1991). *The four little dragons.* Cambridge, MA: Harvard University Press.

Wu, D. Y. H. (1996). Chinese childhood socialization. In M. H. Bond (Ed.), *The handbook of Chinese psychology.* Hong Kong: Oxford University Press.

PART V

The Promotion of Physical Activity Participation

Having examined the current deplorable state of physical activity participation by Hong Kong children as referenced in Part II, the consequences thereof in Part III, and the likely conditions responsible for it in Part IV, we now turn to the subject of possible solutions to the problem in this section.

In Chapter 12, Jim Dickinson reviews the health consequences of poor life style habits and discusses strategies to remedy the situation in four domains of life: work, transport, domestic duties and leisure time. He argues for a concerted effort by agencies across a range of fields. Home, school, urban planning, parks and recreation services, the medical community, all should collaborate in efforts to change the physical activity participatory behaviours of the public. A wealth of examples of measures to encourage physical activity is provided.

In Chapter 13, Amy Ha and Graham Fishburne state the extent of inactivity and unhealthy diets and their heath implications in both Hong Kong and Canada, and focus on school physical education as both a contributing factor and a possible future solution. A series of studies examining some aspects of physical education and the effect of interventions is presented along with a case for a change in focus for physical education to one emphasizing the development of an active lifestyle.

In the final chapter, Koenraad Lindner once again points to school physical education as the obvious mechanism for bringing about changes in the physical activity participation habits of Hong Kong children. The physical education curriculum as it was in the past, as it currently is in most places, and what it should be in the future, is discussed in this chapter, which closes with the observation that such reform ideas are now beginning to be adopted in various places around the world, including Hong Kong.

CHAPTER *12*

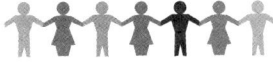

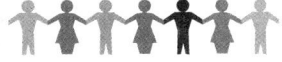

Some Possible Strategies to Combat Sedentary Lifestyles of Hong Kong Youth

Jim Dickinson

Introduction

The findings described in the previous chapters demonstrate that a major problem of sedentary lifestyles is arising in Hong Kong as in other developed and developing societies around the world (World Health Organization, 2002). The findings in this book concentrate on children, but are consistent with data across all age groups. As elsewhere (Bouchard, 2000), the problems are due to a mixture of too little physical activity and a diet that has been modernised, moving to white rice and high fat foods with relatively little vegetable and fruit content. These have resulted in increasing prevalence of obesity, and a particularly Hong Kong phenomenon of a substantial proportion of people who are not grossly obese, but whose body composition contains a high proportion of fat because of low bone and muscle proportion, which in turn are due to very low activity levels.

Even more rapidly than Western countries, Hong Kong has changed from a society in which physical activity was an exhausting part of daily life for the vast majority of the population, to one where most of the population has no need for even moderate physical exertion at any time. Across each of the four domains of daily life: Work, Transport, Domestic duties and Leisure time, the amount of physical exertion has changed enormously. Even childcare, housework, gardening, and home maintenance, which provide activity in less crowded societies are minimal in the small apartments of Hong Kong, particularly since Hong Kong people with large living space often delegate these tasks to foreign house-maids. In high temperatures and humidity for most of the year, energetic movement such as brisk walking becomes undesirable, since the sweating thus produced is socially unpleasant at close quarters. Thus many visitors find that the speed of Hong Kong crowds is frustratingly slow, so that even walking provides less cardiovascular exercise than in other countries where the accustomed pace is faster.

While obesity levels in Hong Kong are nowhere near those in many Western countries, the fear is that it may soon catch up. In the United States, the rise among schoolchildren has been dramatic in recent years (Bouchard, 2000). Now is the time for Hong Kong to prevent this, rather than wait until it is too late.

Outcomes

The most commonly observed adverse health consequences of obesity are diabetes and heart disease, but other health problems also are on the increase. Table 1 shows the range of diseases that are caused by this combination of poor diet and exercise associated with obesity. Obesity from childhood increases these risks, and lowers the age at which the disease becomes manifest. In the USA McGinnis and Foege (1993) calculated that 50% of all deaths are caused by preventable illness, and 14% are due to diet and exercise, second in number only to 19% of tobacco-caused deaths. In Hong Kong, where smoking was, and is now, less prevalent than in the US, the proportion of deaths due to diet and inactivity may be higher. In addition to these specific diseases, obese people are more likely to a recover slower after operations, and are often susceptible to chronic skin infections, varicose veins and leg ulcers. The costs of treating these diseases, and the loss of productivity are enough to make investing in change worthwhile, let alone the human cost of the event.

Approaches to solutions

Each of the four domains of daily life described above provides

Table 1. Diseases caused or exacerbated by inactivity and high fat diet, and their consequences

Cardiovascular	Type 2 Diabetes
• High blood pressure • High blood cholesterol • Congestive heart failure • Ischaemic heart disease mortality, morbidity from cardiac failure, and arrhythmias • Stroke	• Renal failure • Ischaemic cardiovascular disease • Peripheral vascular disease • Peripheral neuritis
Respiratory • Obstructive sleep apnea • Breathlessness • Obesity-related respiratory problems	Digestive • Gall bladder stones • Gall bladder disease
Cancer • Colon • Breast • Prostate • Endometrial • Kidney	Musculo-skeletal • Osteoarthritis • Back pain • Osteoporosis • Falls in the elderly
Psychological disorders • Depression and anxiety • Eating disorders • Distorted body image • Low self-esteem	Reproductive • Poor female reproductive health (e.g., menstrual irregularities, infertility, irregular ovulation) • Complications of pregnancy (e.g., gestational diabetes, gestational hypertension, preeclampsia • Complications in operative delivery (e.g., Caesarian sections)
Health-related quality of life	

Sources: US Department of Health and Human Services (1996; 2001)

opportunities for change. Physical activity is related to needs and opportunities for personal exertion or using mechanical assistance. Activities are complex social behaviours that are related to beliefs across several generations beyond social class lines. These are being modified and to some extent homogenised into the modern media-disseminated

Hong Kong culture. The choices for personal enjoyment are learned, and also depend on opportunities available to each individual within the culture and society, which in turn depend on income, leisure time, and where people live. This complex mixture cannot be solved by one simple approach. Interventions must be developed in a range of fields, and pushed forward simultaneously.

The "medical approach" is important: it provides treatment of the casualties as disease develops, or through screening for high-risk rates. In this case, the medical approach involves detection and treatment of hypertension, coronary heart disease, diabetes, and high blood cholesterol or worse, heart attacks, strokes etc. In the past, doctors have not regarded obesity and inactivity as "risk factors" and adequate research is unavailable on this subject (Campbell, Waters, OMeara, et al., 2002; Summerbell, Ashton, Campbell, et al., 2002). Consequently their education and attention focuses more on biochemistry, genetics and drug treatments than on diet and exercise, as shown by any medical textbook [Sung, Li, Sanderson, & Woo, 1998] or conference on diabetes and hypertension. This is changing gradually (Bauman & Egger, 2000). In Western countries with well-developed primary medical care such as Britain, much prevention and early treatment work is done in front line health care. Starfield (1998) has shown that health outcomes are better in countries where primary care has a greater role, and others point out that where prevention in medical care is specifically rewarded, it is better performed. In Hong Kong, primary medical care is poorly resourced, and unsystematic in its approach, with little encouragement for exemplary preventive care. This is slowly improving, with the development of better training and resourcing of primary care, but still, both in the public and private sectors, primary care doctors focus mainly on acute and chronic illness not on health promotion.

But even primary medical care usually occurs too late. The pathological changes start long before patients cross thresholds for medical recognition and intervention. Worse, medical approaches through individual consultations encouraging behaviour change, weight loss, and drug treatments are relatively expensive yet only partly effective. If it can be done, primary prevention is much better. Geoffrey Rose (1992) pointed out that when a whole population has raised values of cardiac risk factors, much greater effect would occur by regarding the whole population as "at risk", rather than by targeting only a specific fraction which measures above the defined cut-off levels. As he points out: "It makes little sense to expect individuals to behave differently to their peers; it is more appropriate to seek a general change in behavioural norms and in the circumstances which facilitate adoption" (Rose, 1992, cited by World Health Organization, 2002, p. 24). Consequently the best approach is a strategy that involves the whole society and across all age groups. Each segment of society will require a different approach relevant to its own needs and immediate concerns, yet well coordinated to ensure that they are complimentary rather than competing.

A systematic review by Trost, Owen, Bauman, et al. [2002] summarises results from over 300 studies of the correlates of adults' participation in physical activity (Table 2). Most are cross sectional studies. The strength of evidence is not as good as we would like, but they are fairly consistent. Whereas not all the studies will apply well in Hong Kong, they give a framework to think about what can be changed to increase the chance of physical activity. Most particularly, this review shows that multiple factors to support or block activity may be operating simultaneously. Thus our goals must be to understand, reduce barriers, and ultimately to increase encouraging factors.

It is notable that attitudes to exercise, knowledge of health benefits from exercise, and the perceived value of exercise outcomes in reducing susceptibility to illness play little role in actual activity. The perception that exercising requires high intensity and effort has negative effects. While more works needs to be done on this subject, particularly in Hong Kong, these findings suggest that special efforts are needed to focus on the elderly, those with lower educational levels and social class, to include women, and encourage obese individuals. We need to help people to enjoy exercise and its immediate benefits in terms of feeling good, to overcome what people regard as the barriers to exercise, to encourage doctors to recommend exercise and friends and families to encourage one another to do so. We have to make sure that facilities suitable for all groups of people are available within a short distance of each household, and varied to be suitable

Table 2. Factors positively associated with leisure time physical activity in adults

Demographic and biological	Psychological, cognitive and emotional
• Younger age • Higher social class, education, income • Male gender • Normal weight	• Enjoyment of exercise • Expecting benefits • Intending to exercise, perceived health and fitness • No barriers and have enough time • Better psychological health and body image
Behavioural attributes and skills	Social and cultural factors
• Activity during adult life • High quality diet • Skills to cope with barriers to exercise • Non-smoker	• Physician influence • Social support from friends, peers, spouse, family
Physical environment	
• Access to facilities, actual and perceived • Seeing others exercising	• Climate / season • Urban environment
• Enjoyable surroundings, satisfaction with facilities	

Source: selected and adapted from Trost et al. (2002)

for all seasons. Exercise facilities should be enjoyable, so that people can watch and participate in rural and urban environments.

The value of these suggestions is reinforced by a systematic review of interventions conducted in Australia primarily by medical practitioners. Suggestions by doctors to their inactive patients to increase exercise can be effective particularly when embedded in a multifaceted community-wide approach (Smith, Merom, Harris, & Bauman, 2003). Thus, a range of sectors needs to be involved including the local government, transport, urban development and planning, education, sport and recreation and parks services.

All four domains, Work, Transport, Home and Leisure must be considered. It is better to use the term "physical activity" rather than "exercise", since the latter has the connotation of leisure activity, while the former covers all fields. The Australian physical activity guidelines express a useful approach. (Box 1).

Box 1.

National Physical Activity Guidelines for Australia
• Think of movement as an opportunity, not an inconvenience
• Be active every day in as many ways as you can
• Put together at least 30 minutes of moderate intensity physical activity on most, preferably all, days
• If you can, also enjoy some regular vigorous exercise for extra health and fitness

http://www.health.gov.au/pubhlth/strateg/active/links.htm

Much of the total daily activity requirements can also come from ordinary daily work and household care. The few people who still do major physical work such as labourers or deliverymen are seldom obese, and have no need for leisure sports. Many ordinary people can also exert themselves considerably during their daily routine. Some do so because they walk long distances instead of using public transport, or even in the interchanges between different modes of transportation. This has been developed as a major strategy — urging people to walk some part of their journey to or from work or by getting off their buses a few stops earlier.

Hong Kong is justly proud of its public transport network. However, it is almost too convenient. In particular, school buses routinely take children from the door of their home to the door of the school. It has been shown that children who walk to school may spend as much energy doing so as on all other activities combined. Perhaps support for school buses need to be reduced, so as to make them less convenient, that children will walk more!

Children and inactivity

Physical inactivity starts at a young age. Outside visitors are surprised that despite the density of housing, the noises of children at play are seldom heard in Hong Kong housing estates. Toddlers and preschool children are already limited in their movements, in part because the surroundings of many housing estates are paved with concrete with sharp edges and steps, so that children running around can easily be hurt. But movement and activity is not encouraged even where it is safe. Most housing complexes have small play gyms that would exhaust the interest and imagination of small children before exhausting them physically. Most Hong Kong children are enrolled from age three or four into preschools. Unlike the original kindergartens, which emphasised active learning, movement and play, most of these preschools place a premium on children sitting quietly and working at desks. Many have no outside play area at all. The foods provided are mostly unhealthy (Lau, 2002).

Clearly, change must happen at this early age. Parents and caregivers must be encouraged to allow vigorous physical activity at least outside the household. But in order to do so, the architects of housing estates should provide safe play areas that encourage running, chasing, climbing, ball playing and other activities for young children.

In primary and secondary schools there is a possibility of change. That too, is limited by infrastructure. Given the small area available for each school, facilities for sport are far more limited than in most similarly wealthy societies. Changing rooms with showers are absent from most schools. The fear of exercise during severe air pollution periods worsens the problem. The evidence that regular moderate physical activity does not hinder academic learning may allay the fears that examination results will drop as a result of greater physical activity (Lindner, 1999, 2002). However, there will always be a limit to the amount of physical activity possible through school-based programmes. Ways must be found to encourage and increase the leisure-time physical activity of children and adolescents, so it becomes a "normal" part of their lives, so that enjoyment of and participation in physical activity carries on into adulthood.

Daily activities

In common with other major cities of the world, most Hong Kong people work or live in high-rise buildings, where elevators are necessary. They occupy the centre of the lobby and floor plan in most buildings. Residents usually wait a long time for elevators, even to change one or two floors. Part of the problem is that in most buildings the stairs are primarily designed as fire escapes, and are hidden away. If building design were changed to make stairs more easily accessible and inviting to use, many more people could be encouraged to use them for short vertical distances. In doing so, they would reduce over crowding, and walk themselves to fitness: while often getting to their destination faster. Similarly, subway stations, shopping centres, and similar public places could place greater emphasis on stairs than they do at present. They should be a central feature preferable to escalators or elevators. In the UK and the USA, programmes to encourage using stairs are successful and have added substantially to the total amount of daily activity for many people (The Community Guide, 2002), although the impact may be brief, with regression back to routine behaviour unless continuing programmes are emphasized.

Leisure

The types of leisure time physical activity that will best suit Hong Kong people need to be considered. For many, the ideal place for exercise is now the gym, with air conditioning, special clothing and complex equipment. Others think in terms of organised team sport, with regular bookings required for special facilities for practice and games. Neither of these is adequate for the vast majority of the population who cannot afford the cost, nor have regular time available. Emphasis must be placed on activities suited to the limited flatland space of Hong Kong and the prevailing weather. They must use simple, cheap equipment affordable for the majority of Hong Kong people and that can easily be stored in their limited living space. For example many people have insufficient room to store a bicycle. Permanent equipment that is vandal-proof and can be left in place through any weather is important. Lights are necessary for night use, when temperatures are lower, and more people have leisure time. Public education needs to focus on physical activity that requires no organization, and can be done casually, either alone or with a small and variable group of friends. Special consideration should be given to women who have doubts about activities that may display their bodies in public or cause sweating. This is a problem in Western societies (Wen, 2002), but in the Hong

Kong Chinese tradition, the ideal woman is supposed to be delicate, not strong nor athletic in her built.

Basketball is one classic sport suitable for these conditions, and its feasibility and popularity is shown in the courts (used largely by groups of young men) dotted around housing estates. Water sports, such as water polo would also seem appropriate, though more difficult in practice because of the excessively bureaucratic rules in public swimming complexes (compared to other countries).

Walking along the waterfronts and in the hills is also a good activity. People are more likely to walk if the environment is enjoyable, the location is convenient and the company is appropriate (Humpel, Owen, & Leslie, 2002). A valuable feature of Hong Kong is that the centre of the city and many town centres in the New Territories are well designed with elevated walkways that make movement much easier and safer than on the streets. Given the dense population, this programme needs much greater expansion. For example, walkways going through the whole length of the city would reduce street-level congestion, avoid traffic fumes, and provide an enjoyable route for people to walk instead of using transport.

Countryside walking is very popular, especially on Hong Kong Island, where a network of paths around the peaks has been well developed. A dweller can easily get onto these paths and enjoy their walk within a very short distance of home. In Kowloon and the New Territories, the development of such pathways is much less advanced. For example from Shatin, while there are many tracks into the hills, nearly all require a steep uphill climb and very few are paved or constructed along the contours in a way that suits those who are not very agile. The waterfront walks are used, but seldom crowded, not surprising given the unappealing smell of the Shing Mun Channel. Yet the Tai Po waterfront park is very busy, showing that when good facilities are available, they will be used. There are many rural pathways into country parks, but most people without cars can only use them on weekends. More facilities are needed closer to home. Although much of the harbour front has been used for port activities, there are still large stretches where easier and better access to waterfront paths can be developed to encourage more people to walk. Perhaps Hong Kong needs a waterfront route to match the Maclehose Trail.

Sporting activities that require relatively large ground area per participant, that run for long periods of time, a great deal of training, and detailed organization for large teams are not suitable for Hong Kong. These sports include many Western games such as football in most of its variants, cricket, and hockey. Golf is far too expensive for most Hong Kong people. Badminton is better than tennis, since it requires less space per game and less strength to get started. Water sports should be more common given the climate; however, boat sports are only advisable in locations where the water is not too contaminated. The large and expensive equipment makes sailing unaffordable for most people, though windsurfing, canoeing, kayaking and rowing should be better developed. Cycling is possible on the few flat areas, but more cycling paths are needed since road cycling is dangerous on Hong Kong's narrow roads. In the past twenty years, Germany and The Netherlands have changed policies to encourage walking and cycling on short journeys, by providing opportunities that are both pleasant and safe. Separation from motorized traffic and measures to slow motor vehicles has made walking and cycling safer (Pucher & Dijkstra, 2003). Hong Kong needs to think flexibly about how to apply similar ideas.

The older generation of Chinese adults has a good legacy of keeping fit through activity. This is demonstrated by the large number of participants in the early morning walk or *Tai Chi* practice, either alone or within classes. This is commendable, though still not enough people are participating. Worse, many think that such flexibility and stretching exercise is enough to make a difference to their metabolic state. They need encouragement to do aerobic activity such as walking as well. This can be done in groups through the elderly clubs found in each district, and in association with the elderly health services.

Public behaviour change

How can changes in attitude and behaviour be encouraged? There are many possible entry points to changing health-related societal behaviour. We must inquire what behaviours should be changed, for which population groups, and who is best placed to assist that process of change.

Increase in physical activity can reduce body weight, fat proportion (Irwin,Yasui, Ulrich, et al., 2003); and lower blood pressure (Whelton, Chin, Xin, & He, 2002). It can reduce cardiovascular risk and slow or reverse the development of diabeties (Diabetes Prevention Program Research Group, 2002). Activity improves control in those who have become diabetic, (Lam, 2002) reduces symptoms in osteoarthritis, and progression of osteoporosis. Thus moderate level of physical activity by people of all ages prevents future health problems, reduces existing ones and thereby lowers total death risk [Lee, Hsieh, & Paffenbarger, 1995).

Clearly, while this book has focussed mainly on school-age children, the problem encompasses most of society. In families where the expectations and modelling of behaviour are shared by at least two and often three generations, it is unlikely that interventions addressed to children will be effective unless the rest of their family can be included and their ideas are changed. Thus we need to consider how to change all together.

Different categories of personal have performed interventions in trials to increase activity. Any can be effective if the staff have enough time and are focussed on the needs of the target group [Eakin, Glasgow, & Riley, 2000). However, while it may seem to be a sound principle to have medical practitioners prescribe and encourage activity, routine advice given by doctors whose focus and priorities are often elsewhere is unlikely to be effective (Hillsdon, Thorogood, White, & Foster, 2002; Task Force on Community Preventive Services, 2003).

An initial approach to tackle this problem was "Health Education" where for nurses to give lectures in schools. They put up posters and distribute campaign materials in public places while giving "health education" talks to community groups. The Hong Kong Department of Health has been performing this type of programme. While it initially focussed on more directly health-related matters such as cleanliness, immunisation, antenatal and childrearing issues it has diversified, to include the need for exercise as one of its many goals in recent years. However, given limited funding and multiple missions, this kind of programme will never be adequate. Furthermore, while such methods work in poorly educated societies with a coercive-style government, in a sophisticated modern society such as Hong Kong, they have limited impact in changing behaviour.

Simple delivery of information is seldom effective. In the field of school smoking education well-planned anti-smoking programmes often have minimal effect (Thomas, Trost, Owen, et al., 2002). Thus much more subtle and sophisticated methods may be needed, using multiple different approaches. The perception of social acceptability, cigarette price changes, education and advertising campaigns help to reduce smoking rates, but these changes are slow. Modern health promotion incorporates multiple modes to transmit information, and to articulate a change in beliefs and behaviours, while evaluating to ensure that each component is effective.

The United States Task Force on Community Preventive Services (2002) has assessed the evidence for these approaches to physical activity. Table 3 summarizes its current assessment of the evidence for different types of intervention. Well-designed media campaigns to increase physical activity can work.

Some of these recommendations, especially the negative ones, may appear surprising, but much of the research has been performed in the United States, with some in Australia, the United Kingdom and elsewhere. Applying the findings to Hong Kong may not be possible as it is a very different society, and careful evaluation is needed to ensure that the data apply.

This review left out workplace programmes. There are many of these, and various businesses have calculated that the value of a healthy workforce is worth the cost and effort of a workplace fitness programme. The Canadian Physical Activity Guide website gives examples of savings, and presents a "business case" for active healthy living programmes at work (Canada's Physical Activity Guide, 2003).

Role models are important in showing the population that activity is good, and behaviour to be emulated. The medical profession was convinced that smoking causes disease, and many changed their behaviour, so that finding a smoking doctor is now very difficult in many countries. Such unanimous behaviour change by those who are perceived as having solid background knowledge gives far greater credibility to the message. For physical activity, role modelling by the Hong Kong medical profession is less clear. Dr Lo Wing Lok has always emphasised participation in physical activity, for example the annual Trail walker, and the HK Medical Association has a variety of sporting

Table 3. Approaches to increasing physical activity

Informational approaches
• Strongly recommended
Community–wide campaigns to promote physical activity
• Recommended
Point of decision prompts to encourage use of stairs
• Insufficient evidence
Mass media campaigns
Classroom-based health education focussed on information provision
Behavioural and social approaches
• Strongly recommended
School-based Physical education
Social support interventions in community settings
Individually-adapted health behaviour interventions
• Insufficient evidence
College-based health education and PE
Classroom-based health education focussed on reducing television
viewing and videogame playing
Family–base support
Environmental and Policy approaches to increasing Physical activity
• Strongly recommended
Creation of or enhanced access to places for physical activity
combined with information outreach activities

Source: Task Force on Community Preventive Services (2002)

and fun activities, but levels of involvement are low. Moreover, while hospitals are now smoke free, they do not encourage physical activity or good eating patterns by the students or staff who often must stay on site for long periods. A former Dean of Medicine at The Chinese University, Professor Sydney Chung runs marathons, and has encouraged the setup of an exercise room for residential students and "fun runs" for members of the faculty, but few participate as yet. It appears that doctors who are from or educated overseas, or who have become acculturated to Western ideas are more likely to participate. Ordinary community doctors, who work long hours, like their patients, tend not to exercise much. Mechanisms need to be found so that they themselves change their behaviour, as exemplars for the population. Teachers are also important role models for school children, so they are an important target for behaviour change activity. Some may argue that it is difficult to change deeply embedded Chinese beliefs about physical activity. That may be true, but the glory of Hong Kong is the rapid adaptation of its people to a modern industrial society. When Hong Kong people settle overseas, they rapidly adapt to the environment there. Indeed some of the most active Chinese in Hong Kong are those who have brought back these habits after returning from their study abroad.

Reducing the barriers to available facilities is important. A slogan used in some campaigns was "make active choices the easy choices" Given the extreme limitations on space in most residential areas, and the extended hours of work for Hong Kong people, good facilities in each area need to be available. Thus schoolyards should be redesigned so that community members can use them in non-school hours. Facilities such as playing fields and swimming pools need to be open from early morning until late at night. Which facilities are used for formal activities, they should still be available to informal groups. For example, swimming pool complexes should arrange that some lanes can be used by swimmers who want to exercise vigorously, while other parts are used for unstructured play. The municipal sports complexes need to reconsider the patterns of closure at meal times that seem to be more for the convenience of staff than that of the public. In other countries many office workers exercise during their mid-day break or in the early evening, just when Hong Kong facilities usually close. Sporting facilities should be used, and if they wear out quickly, that should be regarded as evidence of their value, rather than cost.

Conclusion

Hong Kong is not alone in needing to combat sedentary lifestyles. The United States, Australia, Canada, United Kingdom and many European countries are trying to make similar changes. They are all learning as they go along, evaluating and testing various approaches. Hong Kong should also participate in this process.

Societal change cannot be quick, but must start as soon as possible, to encompass the whole of the society. Schools are one portal to start.

Well-trained physical education teachers produced by the universities are good, but the number is limited and they are not always in a good position to make major changes. However, recently the Healthy Schools Programme is educating school teachers in a range of actions to improve health in populations through a postgraduate diploma course. This programme is funded by the Quality Education Fund (Lee, Tsang, Lee, & To, 2003). Physical activity is one component of this course, and a major topic for projects that participants select. Over time, these graduates may provide evidence for selecting promising interventions that can be more widely applied. Liaison needs to be developed between these teachers and the existing cadre of physical education teachers.

Policies in regard to urban planning are also needed. Danneberg, Jackson, Frumkin, et al. (2003) describe changes for the US, but since Hong Kong starts from a different situation, it will need to move forward in subtly different ways. This will require changing the rules for architects and developers, town planning consideration, and better design for parks and recreation facilities. In Australia, changed attractiveness of walking routes, including such factors as shade and the lack of vehicle traffic, was related to how much people walk, both for recreation and for transport. (Giles-Corti, & Donovan, 2003)

An example of success has come from the dietary field. Here a small group of activists has combined, using local evidence, to encourage the health and education departments to recognise their role as exemplars in providing of nutritious food in schools. The healthy tuckshop programme has changed the type of foods available for purchase, while educating teachers, children and parents about what they should expect from healthy foods. Change in practice occurs only slowly. Similar approaches are possible in the exercise field.

If thought through critically, with more attention paid to popular mass activity, rather than only to elite groups, a substantial change in population activity level is possible. This will require gaining the attention of societal leaders, whose focus is understandably placed on dealing with the economic rather than the physical, emotional and mental health of the region. Making change will require multiple and diversified approaches, through lobby groups, producing information that is salient to decision-makers, and suggesting solutions that will not be too costly. However, the economic case for more physical activity is strong, based on health care cost alone. For example, drugs for diabetes and high cholesterol are one of the largest budget items for the Hospital Authority. Small expenditure could create substantial improvements. Campaigns can also use social heroes such as Lee Lai Shan as exemplars. Also, Hong Kong could encourage community level sport leagues that would bring many neighbourhood groups or friendly teams together. Such programmes would increase the level of general activity, and Hong Kong might even build on this base to perform well in international competitions.

References

Bauman, A. & Egger, G. (2000). The dawning of a new era for physical inactivity as a health risk factor. *Australian & New Zealand Journal of Medicine, 30*, 65–7, 2000.

Bouchard, C. (Ed.) (2000). *Physical activity and obesity.* Champaign, IL.: Human Kinetics.

Campbell, K., Waters, E., O'Meara, S., Kelly, S., & Summerbell, C. (2003). Interventions for preventing obesity in children. *Cochrane Database of Systematic Reviews, 3.*

Canada's Physical Activity Guide (2003). http://www.hc-sc.gc.ca/hppb/paguide/ (accessed October 11 2003).

Danneberg, A. L., Jackson, R. J., Frumkin, H., Scheiber, R. A., Pratt, M., Kochitzky, C., & Tilson, H. H. (2003). The impact of community design and land-use. *American Journal of Public Health, 93*, 1500–1508.

Diabetes Prevention Program Research Group (2002). Reduction in the incidence of type 2 diabetes with lifestyle intervention or metformin. *New England Journal of Medicine, 4346*, 393–403.

Eakin, E. G., Glasgow, R. E., & Riley, K. M. (2000). Review of primary care-based physical activity intervention studies. Effectiveness and implications for practice and future research. *Journal of Family Practice, 49*, 158–68.

Giles-Corti, B., & Donovan, R. J. (2003). Relative influences of individual, social environmental, and physical environmental correlates of walking. *American Journal of Public Health, 93*, 1583–1589.

Hillsdon, M., Thorogood, M., White, I., & Foster, C. (2002). *International Journal of Epidemiology, 31*, 808–15.

Humpel, N., Owen, N., & Leslie, E. (2002). Environmental factors associated with adults' participation in physical activity. *American Journal of Preventive Medicine, 22(3)*, 188–199.

Irwin, M. L., Yasui, Y., Ulrich, C. M., Bowden, D., Rudolph, R. E., Schwartz, S. R., Yukawa, M., Aiello, E., Potter, J. D., & McTiernan, A. (2003). Effect of exercise on total and intra-abdominal fat body in postmenopausal women: A randomised controlled trial. *Journal of the American Medical Association, 289*, 3223–3230.

Lam, A. (2002). *Trial of a new education program for diabetic patients.* M.Phil. thesis, The Chinese University of Hong Kong.

Lau, L. (2001). *Diet and lifestyles among the preschool children.* M. Phil. thesis, The Chinese University of Hong Kong.

Lee, I. M., Hsieh, C. C., & Paffenbarger, R. S. Jr. (1995). Exercise intensity and longevity in men. The Harvard Alumni Health Study. *Journal of the American Medical Association, 273*, 1179–1184.

Lee, A., Tsang, C., Lee, S. H., To, C. Y. (2003). A comprehensive "Healthy Schools Programme" to promote school health: The Hong Kong experience in joining the efforts of health and education sectors. *Journal of Epidemiology and Community Health, 57*, 174–177

Lindner, K. J. (1999). Sport participation and perceived academic performance of school children and youth. *Pediatric Exercise Science, 10*, 129–143.

Lindner, K. J. (2002). The activity participation — academic performance relationship revisited: Perceived and actual performance, and the effect of banding (academic tracking). *Pediatric Exercise Science, 14*, 155–169.

McGinnis, J. A. M., & Foege, W. H. (1993). Actual causes of death in the United States. *Journal of the American Medical Association, 270*, 207–212.

National Physical Activity Guidelines for Australia. http://www.health.gov.au/pubhlth/strateg/active/links.htm (accessed October 12 2003)

Pucher, J., & Dijkstra, (2003). Promoting safe walking and cycling to improve public health: Lessons from the Netherlands and Germany. *American Journal of Public Health, 93*, 1509–1516.

Rose G. (1992). *The strategy of preventive medicine.* Oxford: Oxford University Press.

Smith, B. J., Merom, D., Harris, P., & Bauman, A.E. (2003). Do physical activity interventions to promote physical activity work? A systematic review of the literature. Melbourne: National Institute of Clinical Studies. Available at http//www.cpah.unsw.edu.au/NICS.pdf (accessed Oct 11 2003)

Starfield (1998). *Primary care: Balancing health needs, services and technology.* New York, NY: Oxford University Press.

Summerbell, C. D., Ashton, V., Campbell, K. J., Edmunds, L., Kelly, R., & Waters, E. (2002). Interventions for treating obesity in children. *Cochrane Databases of Systematic Reviews, 3.*

Sung, J. Y., Li, P. K. T., Sanderson, J. E., & Woo, J. (1998*). Textbook of clinical medicine for Asia.* Hong Kong: The Chinese University of Hong Kong Press.

Task Force on Community Preventive Services (2002). Recommendations to increase physical activity in communities. *American Journal of Preventive Medicine, 22*

The Guide to Community Preventive Services (2003). *Point of decision prompts to encourage use of stairs. Evidence summary table.* http://www.thecommunity guide.org/pa/default.htm (accessed 12 October 2003).

Thomas, R., Trost, S. G., Owen, N., Bauman, A. E., Sallis, J. F., & Brown, W. (2002). Correlates of adults' participation in physical activity: Review and update. *Medicine and Science of Sport and Exercise, 34,* 1996–2001.

Trost, S. G., Owen, N., Bauman, A. E., Sallis, J. F., & Brown, W. (2002). Correlates of adults' participation in physical activity: Review and update. *Medicine and Science of Sport and Exercise, 34,* 1996–2001.

US Department of Health and Human Services (1996*). Physical activity and health: A report of the surgeon-general.* Atlanta GA: US Department of Health and Human Services. Centres for Disease Control and Prevention, National Center for Chronic Disease Prevention and Health Promotion.

US Preventive Services Task Force (2003). Behavioural counselling in primary care to promote physical activity: Recommendations and rationale. *American Journal of Nursing, 103,* 101–107.

Wen, L. M., Thomas, M., Jones, H., Orr, N., Moreton, R., King, L., Hawe, P., Bindon, J., Humphries, J., Schicht, K., Corne, S., & Bauman, A. (2002). Promoting physical activity in women: Evaluation of a 2-year community-based intervention in Sydney, Australia. *Health Promotion International, 17,* 127–37.

Whelton, S. P., Chin, A., Xin, X., & He, J. (2002). Effect of aerobic exercise on blood pressure: A meta analysis of randomised controlled trials. *Annals of Internal Medicine, 136,* 493–503.

World Health Organization (2002). *The World Health Report 2002: Reducing risks, promoting healthy life.* Geneva: Author.

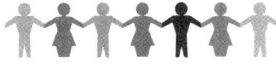

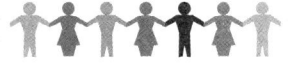

CHAPTER 13

The Role of the School in Promoting Healthy and Active Lifestyles among Hong Kong School Children

Amy Ha and Graham J. Fishburne

Introduction

This chapter discusses the important role school physical education plays in a child's development. A brief review of the financial and human costs associated with physical inactivity is presented to demonstrate the problems associated with physical inactivity and poor eating habits. To help combat physical inactivity a case is made for quality programmes of school physical education. If children are to engage in active healthy lifestyles they will need the knowledge, skills, and attitudes necessary for successful participation in physical activity. Hence school physical education will have a vital role to play if the current trend among children, youth and adults of sedentary unhealthy lifestyles, which is seen in most countries of the world today, is to be changed. The school and the education system play a vital role in teaching and facilitating the development of the knowledge, skills, and attitudes that facilitate active healthy lifestyles. The potential impact of quality programmes of school physical education on the future health of Hong Kong children, youth and adults is discussed in this chapter.

How Healthy are Our Children?

Sedentary lifestyles among children and youth are quite common in today's technological societies. There are many reasons to sit for hours in front of a computer or television screen. Indeed, with electronic mail and web camera software computer programmes a child no longer has to engage in the physical effort required to visit and play with neighborhood friends as all this can be achieved while sitting in front of a computer screen. Also, labour saving devices abound in today's world. No longer do people have to physically lift the garage door, push a lawnmower, manually open a can, or even walk to the television to change a channel. All of these tasks can be easily achieved through minimal physical effort thanks to advances in technology. But what is the cost of this sedentary lifestyle? Decreased physical fitness and weight gain usually accompany physical inactivity. As a result increases in child obesity rates and increases in child diabetes are two of the major health concerns associated with today's physically inactive lifestyles.

Physical inactivity and its related effects on health can be seen in most countries today. Two countries, Hong Kong and Canada, will be discussed in this chapter to illustrate the common problems faced through inactivity and the poor eating and nutritional habits of young people in today's world.

In Hong Kong the inactivity of young people has been well documented and has become a health concern. As stated, sedentary inactive lifestyles result in poor fitness and health problems. Studies have shown Hong Kong children to be unfit and inactive (Chan, Li, Hong & Leung, 1998; Johns & Ha, 1999; Lindner, 1998). For example, MacFarlane (1997) reported that less than 4% of a group of primary children in Hong Kong were able to maintain light to moderate vigorous physical activity for a designated period of twenty minutes. Johns and Ha (1999) also found that Hong Kong children's active behaviors were extremely limited in both the school and home setting. It is disturbing to note that children in Hong Kong seem to exhibit even lower levels of physical fitness than children from neighbouring countries (Eston, Ingledew, Fu, & Rowlands, 1998; Hatano, Jua, Jiang, Fu, Zhi, & Wei, 1997;).

The children and youth of Canada exhibit behaviours that would appear to be consistent with the trends seen in Hong Kong. A rise in obesity rates, type 2 diabetes, and sedentary lifestyles is the common trend among Canadian children and youth today (Fishburne, McKay, & Berg, 2002).

Diet and Nutrition

It is not only changes in physical activity patterns that have contributed to a decline in children's health. Changes in diet and eating habits also play a large role. In the 2002 opening address of the 12th Commonwealth International Sport Conference Professor Timothy Noakes of the University of Cape Town in South Africa identified changes in our diet and the food options available. He noted that when the 'Big Mac' hamburger was first introduced into MacDonald's restaurants its caloric content was just over 600 calories. For a little extra in money you can now 'super size' your food in many of today's 'fast food' restaurants, meaning larger portions are now available. You can now purchase a Big Mac hamburger meal that contains over 1800 calories — a caloric intake that is often recommended for an entire day. Professor Noakes also pointed out his concern for the health and well-being of our children and youth, noting that despite the rapid internationalization of sport over the past twenty years the benefit of sport and physical activity for the 'masses' has not been realized. He noted that:

> ... *children born in the last 25 years of the 20th century, certainly in the developed world, will be less physically active, less physically fit and probably less healthy than their immediate predecessors. Since there is now good evidence that this must inevitably lead to an increased prevalence of medical problems, especially obesity and diabetes, in later life, the future medical consequences of the growing unfitness of the young members of our populations is alarming. Indeed, the paradox is that those developed countries that are the "best" in international sport have not been spared this effect; in fact, perhaps the opposite applies. (p. 10)*

The physical inactivity and related health concerns predicted by Professor Noakes can be seen in the children and youth of Hong Kong and Canada.

Funding Solutions

Often, when problems occur in society, requests for more money are made to help produce solutions. However, of equal importance is the decision as to 'where' money and resources should be targeted. It should be noted that even though greater amounts of 'money' and 'resources' are being committed toward sport in our societies this does not translate to 'mass' participation. A similar argument can be made in education. We continue to add money and resources to school education and to 'research' best practices to improve the quality of education for our children and youth, yet the reality is that the health and physical well-being of many children continue to deteriorate. Historically physical education has received little emphasis in school education and in recent years the situation has deteriorated even further. While money and resources have been committed to areas such as 'technology,' there has been a decline and a neglect of sport and physical education in the great majority of schools around the world (Hardman & Marshall, 2000). Professor Noakes (2002) makes the claim that commercial interests, including television and the fast food industry, have been aided and abetted by the neglect of physical education in our school systems. This combined effect has made "regular physical activity an increasingly unattractive or less relevant option for children" (p. 10). The 'unattractive' nature of physical activity to young people is now seen in many countries around the world. There is a growing trend among children and youth toward sedentary lifestyles and poor eating habits, and as noted, this trend brings with it potential health consequences. Therefore, a greater research effort must be made to help understand how to make physical activity and school physical education more "attractive" to young people. We need to lure the inactive population of children and youth into regular physical activity. Several Hong Kong studies that are presented in the later part of this chapter have focused their research on this area.

Health Implications of Inactivity

It cannot be overemphasized what problems physical inactivity causes in our societies. At a recent conference in Hong Kong (2002b) the keynote address by Professor Fishburne provided evidence of both the financial and human costs of sedentary inactive lifestyles. He used Canada as an example, and stated that the monetary cost of physical inactivity has been estimated at $2.1 billion Canadian dollars per year in that country. The tragic human cost has been estimated at 21,000 premature deaths per year due directly or indirectly to physical inactivity. These Canadian statistics illustrate vividly the health problems and financial costs that accompany physical inactivity. Hence, physical inactivity patterns and low-fitness levels seen among the Hong Kong children and youth of today is a real cause for concern. If the pattern of physical inactivity among Hong Kong children and youth continues this would provide the foundation for future health problems for the people of Hong Kong with a high financial burden.

Obesity

The concern for the rise in levels of obesity in Hong Kong has been reported in several research studies (Lee, Critchley, Chan, et al., 2000; Leung, Ng., & Lau, 1995; Sung, Yu, Chang, et al., 2002; Woo, Leung, Ho, et al., 1999). The trend in Hong Kong mirrors that of other countries where it is the younger age groups that are starting to gain excess weight. This trend is seen in Canada. Over the past 15 years, the prevalence of obesity has tripled in Canadian children aged 7–13 (Tremblay & Willms, 2000). Why are these younger children gaining weight? Is it solely due to physical inactivity? Or is it due to overeating? Reviewing research over the last 30 years does not support significant increases in energy or kilojoule intake. The cause of obesity does not appear to be overeating. In the majority of cases it appears to be due to a combination of physical inactivity and poor nutritional eating habits. If children do not 'overeat' but eat diets high in fat and then do not 'burn off' the excess calories through physical activity, the fat is stored. Sedentary physical inactivity and poor nutritional eating habits are a recipe for weight problems.

There is research evidence to suggest that overweight children increase their chances of becoming overweight adults if they remain overweight beyond adolescence (Dietz & Gortmaker, 2001). Hence the early school years are a sensitive time when healthy living habits need to be established (or the time when intervention programmes need to be put in place). Clearly, school Physical Education and Health Education become important curricula subjects in the early years of schooling.

Diabetes

Approximately 90% of all cases of diabetes are type 2. Type 2 diabetes is not due to the incorrect supply of insulin produced by the body (type 1), it is a result of the body not being able to use correctly the insulin it produces. As in most countries in the world today, a rise in diabetes has been seen in both Hong Kong (Janus, 1997) and Canada (Fishburne, 2002a). Leung and Lam (2000) reported that physical inactivity is one of the major risk factors associated with diabetes in Hong Kong. Physical inactivity, along with obesity, has also been cited in Canada as a major contributor to diabetes. Physical inactivity and obesity contribute greatly to the onset of Type 2 diabetes. It has been reported that approximately 80% of Canadian people with diabetes are overweight or obese. In 1999 it was estimated that 1.2–1.4 million Canadians 12 years and older suffer from diabetes, with approximately 60,000 new cases diagnosed each year. Diabetes is often termed the 'silent disease' as it often leads to long term complications — heart disease, stroke, kidney failure, limb amputation, cataracts, and glaucoma. As stated, the most recognized triggers for type 2 diabetes are physical inactivity and obesity. The prevalence of diabetes in Canada is predicted to double by 2010.

One of the most worrisome research findings is the 'second generation' consequence of type 2 diabetes. It has been reported that the offspring of parents with non-insulin dependent diabetes often show multiple abnormalities in glucose homeostasis early in life as well as high risk measures of body fatness, hence providing the offspring with a predisposition toward diabetes (Fishburne, 2002b).

Osteoporosis

Osteoporosis is a disease characterized by low bone mass and deterioration of bone tissue. This leads to increased bone fragility and risk of fracture, particularly of the hip, spine and wrist. Osteoporosis is known as the 'silent thief' because bone loss occurs without symptoms. More women suffer from this disease than men. Approximately 1 in 4 women and 1 in 8 men over 50 years of age suffer from osteoporosis. Although the effects of this debilitating bone disease often do not show up until middle age, this disease can strike at any age. The problems associated with osteoporosis can be seen in both Hong Kong and Canada. In Hong Kong, Lau and Cooper (1993) reported that the risk of hip fracture has been increasing in Hong Kong due to habitual non-milk diet (a low calcium diet) and physical inactivity. In Canada, the cost of treating osteoporosis and the fractures it causes has been estimated to be $1.3 billion dollars each year. Long term hospital and chronic care account for the majority of these costs. Without effective action on osteoporosis prevention and treatment strategies, it is estimated that over the next 25 years Canada will spend at least $32.5 billion dollars treating osteoporotic fractures (Fishburne, 2002a). Given the increasing proportion of older people in the Canadian population, these costs will likely rise.

In addition to the financial cost of osteoporosis there is the dreadful human cost. The reduced quality of life for those with osteoporosis is enormous. Osteoporosis can result in disfigurement, lowered self-esteem, reduction or loss of mobility, decreased independence, permanent disability, and premature death. Bone fractures as a result of osteoporosis can be devastating. There are approximately 25,000 hip fractures in Canada each year. Seventy percent of these fractures are osteoporosis related. Hip fractures result in death in up to 20 percent of cases, and disability in 50 percent of those who survive. More women die each year as a result of osteoporosis fractures than from breast and ovarian cancer combined (Fishburne, 2002b).

Creating Change in Physical Activity Behaviour

Clearly, changing sedentary physically inactive lifestyles is a challenge that needs to be met. A number of research studies have been conducted to investigate the impact of intervention programmes designed to elicit behaviour change and to provide insights toward programme change. For example, a number of studies have been undertaken in Hong Kong by Ha and her colleagues at the Chinese University of Hong Kong. A brief review of the findings from several of these studies provides important information and insights for changes in Hong Kong.

Perceptions of physical education learning environment of Hong Kong children (Ha, Pang & Cheung, 2004)

The first study reviewed here considered Hong Kong children's perceptions of their school 'physical education' learning environment. Participants (N = 1406), aged from 12 to 15 years, were Hong Kong secondary students and included 698 boys and 708 girls. A Physical Education Learning Environment Scale (PELES) was used to measure student perceptions of their physical education learning environment. Findings from this study showed that boys often attributed their success to effort and ability (task orientation) rather than winning and competition (ego orientation). Such a phenomenon was also supported by the results of perceived competitiveness. When examining the dimension of perceived competitiveness, it was found that younger boys tended to focus on competing and winning, while girls showed less interest in this dimension regardless of their age. Overall, boys scored significantly higher than girls at all ages in this dimension ($p < .05$). In contrast, older girls scored significantly higher than boys on perceived threat ($p < .05$). The findings for this study indicated that girls tend to have less confidence in their own ability in sports, especially as they grow older. Such findings also support the notion that girls have less interest in physical education due to their low self-perception and a lack of self-confidence in physical activities. Clearly, physical educators should continuously make efforts to modify their programmes, their instructional approaches and sports equipment, in order to attract and motivate female students to participate in and enjoy regular physical exercise (See also chapters by Johns & Vertinsky and by Lindner in this volume).

Rope-skipping and a health intervention programme to improve physical activity (Ha, Wong, Chan, & Morris, 2002)

Exercises that emphasize less competition or skill components may be more appropriate to help motivate more children to engage in movement. Rope skipping can be used in such a way. Rope skipping, at a low basic skill level, can be used in a non-competitive manner. A recent study adopted a school population-based approach with the purpose to determine whether or not an 8-week physical education programme with an emphasis on rope skipping and health education could improve students' fitness levels, increase their knowledge of health concepts, and produce positive feelings about physical activity. One thousand four hundred and sixteen children aged 9–14 participated into this project on a volunteer basis. Results of the study indicated that after the intervention programme the experimental groups showed significantly greater improvement in the skipping cardiovascular endurance test compared with a control group. Also, questionnaire responses suggested that children involved in the health education programme had a considerably better understanding of general health and nutrition than those of the control group. However, while the response to feelings about physical activity showed that regardless of improvements in skipping performance and improved knowledge about the importance of health and physical activity, there was no indication that students had changed their feelings towards it. The lack of improvement in positive feelings about physical activity could be indicative of the duration of the intervention period. In order to achieve the positive long lasting behavioural changes educators and health officials desire, it is likely that interventions such as the one described in this study will require a considerable length of intervention time before the activity becomes a more permanent part of an individual's lifestyle. Also, school intervention programmes will require social support from outside the school. Successful interventions will need the support of the home and local community, as well as the school to achieve the consistent reinforcement necessary for the behaviour change (Berg & Fishburne, 2002). Only then will educators be able to change the sedentary lifestyles that have become so prevalent in a modern society. Another important key to behaviour change, however, is the quality of teaching. Catering to different learning styles demands that the teacher deliver different teaching formats. For successful learning the teacher must exhibit competency in the delivery of different instructional formats.

Effect of instructional format on appropriate time in motor skills, heart rate intensity and exercise enjoyment of students (Ha, Johns, & Fung, 2001)

This study was undertaken to examine the effects of different instructional fitness formats on student's appropriate motor time, heart rate intensity and exercise pleasure. The participants in this study consisted of 480 Hong Kong junior secondary school students. Three different instructional formats were provided. One approach was considered a traditional fitness model instructional approach. The remaining two models involved emphasizing fitness skill. The only difference in these two instructional approaches was the addition of musical accompaniment throughout the instructional programme. All three approaches proved effective in developing the desired fitness learning outcomes. However, the participants provided a clear indication of their preferred format of instruction in a questionnaire that was administered at the conclusion of the study. They expressed greatest satisfaction when the instructional format was accompanied by music. These results indicate that attention could be paid to the development and delivery of different instructional teaching formats. Catering to student preferences will not only attract, but could also sustain the interest of young people and could lead to a regular participation in exercise programmes.

Students' perspectives of the physical education curriculum in Hong Kong (Ha, Johns & Shiu, 2003)

The purpose of this study was to examine and analyze students' expectations towards the Hong Kong secondary physical education curriculum. Participants (N = 5,283), were randomly selected from twenty-five Hong Kong secondary schools, and were asked to respond to a 10-item questionnaire about their views of their physical education curriculum. Results showed that about one third of the participants would not choose physical education if the programme were offered as an optional subject. Secondary three, four and five (equivalent to grades 8, 9, and 10) students were the most critical of current activity units. Although both male and female students ranked fitness and skill domains as the top priority among the various learning objectives, female students did not wish to be assessed in these areas. Male students favoured soccer, basketball, handball, fitness and Chinese Kung-fu, while female students preferred volleyball, tennis, badminton, games and creative dance. Over three-fourths of the participants suggested students' opinions should be considered when teachers plan their programme. In order to encourage greater interest in physical activity, respondents in this study requested that new activities should be added to the existing curriculum. Recognizing student's needs and interests could lead to greater participation and adherence to regular physical activity.

Teachers' perceptions of in-service teacher training to support curriculum change in physical education: The Hong Kong experience (Ha, Lee, Chan & Sum, 2004)

Addressing student preferences and providing opportunities for input is obviously key to improving physical activity patterns among Hong Kong students. However of equal importance is the area of 'teacher competence' — competence to deliver quality programmes of physical education. Making changes to curricula is important but of equal importance is the professional development of teachers to implement changes. The purpose of the following study was to evaluate the effectiveness of an in-service training programme and to evaluate teachers' receptivity to curriculum change in physical education. One hundred and eighty-three Hong Kong primary school teachers were voluntarily recruited as participants. They were asked to respond to a questionnaire about their receptivity to changes in the current physical education curriculum as well as their views on the effectiveness of a teacher development programme that was organized by the Chinese University of Hong Kong to help in-service these teachers to effectively teach the new curriculum. Results showed that participants felt that in-service training was needed to equip them to implement a physical education programme in line with the new curriculum reform. The in-service training programme was deemed to be practical and effective, bringing about good communication among schoolteachers, educational experts, and government curriculum officers. In terms of their receptivity to curriculum change, the participants generally had positive attitudes to the innovation and showed further support for the change after attending the programme. The role of the principal and the need for school support were felt to be key elements to facilitate the implementation of a new physical education curriculum.

Benefits of an Active Lifestyle Development

A strong case can be made to improve the quality of physical education programmes in schools (Berg & Fishburne, 2002). Many children complete their school education without developing the necessary skills, knowledge, or attitudes to engage in physically active lifestyles. Although new physical education curricula are being introduced into many schools today the lack of teacher accountability in this subject area often leads to poor learning outcomes. Teachers need to realize the important role they can play in the physical development of children. Hong Kong has taken a leadership role in this area. Like many other countries Hong Kong has made changes to its school physical education curricula. The old Primary (1995) and Secondary (1988) physical education curricula had a major emphasis on sport. Improving children's sports skills, fitness, attitudes to physical activity, and aesthetic appreciation of physical movement were the main aims and objectives. Hence, similar to the traditional approaches seen in most countries, school physical education in Hong Kong had a major emphasis on games and sport activities. Catering to individual differences among students and providing alternative types of physical activity including individual activities, were not commonplace. Typically, before the development of the new PE curriculum, the main focus of the school was to place a high importance on the traditional 'academic' subjects, with areas such as health and physical education playing only a minor role in the hierarchy of importance. Basically, physical education was seen as a subject area that was needed to keep children fit and to teach them how to play sports. After 1997, when Hong Kong was returned to China, the HKSAR government determined that education should be a major area of reform. In 1999 the Education Department initiated a review of the existing school curriculum. The first major change was to propose that physical education, art education, and humanities education be included as 'Key Learning Areas' along with Chinese, English, Mathematics, Science, and Information Technology on equal footing in the school curriculum. Physical Education was no longer to be seen as a 'minor' part of a child's education; it is now seen as one of the 'key learning areas' that can play an important role in a child's development. The top-down hierarchy, with physical education at the bottom as a minor subject area, is no longer viewed as being in the best interests of child development.

The second major change was to the aims and objectives of the new physical education curriculum. The emphasis was removed from the 'sport skills' dominance to the view that 'active, healthy lifestyle development' among children is to become the major aim of the new curriculum (Curriculum Development Council, 2002). Teaching children the knowledge, skills, and attitudes to develop and maintain healthy active lifestyles is now the goal of the new physical education curriculum.

The third change, which probably sets Hong Kong apart from other countries that have moved to the new 'active lifestyle development' PE curricula, is the commitment the Hong Kong Education Department has made to effectively implement their new PE curricula and to make teachers accountable for achieving the learning outcomes associated with the new curriculum (Ha, Lee, Chan, & Sum, 2004). Hence 'assessment' plays a major role in the education reform of the PE curriculum. Further, the government has taken on the responsibility, and provided the financial resources, to in-service teachers on how to implement the new Physical Education curriculum. The thrust to make teachers accountable for delivering the new curriculum and achieving the desired learning outcomes has been demanded by the government. However, the government has also taken on the responsibility to 'teach' teachers this should be done. The added commitment to in-service teachers and to provide guidance and help to teachers with 'assessment' procedures so they can more easily show their accountability, is a leadership role that needs to be recognized (Ha, Chan, & Sum, 2003). Not only has the Hong Kong Education Department recognized the important role physical education plays in a child's development, it has developed a new physical education curriculum that will be accompanied by professional development in-service work to help Hong Kong teachers effectively teach and deliver the new curriculum.

Both the school (teachers) and the education system (government) play a vital role in teaching and facilitating the development of the knowledge, skills, and attitudes in children that will be vital for participation in active healthy lifestyles. Working 'together' will increase the likelihood of achieving the educational goals we desire (Ha, Lee, Chan, & Sum, 2004).

Concluding Remarks

This chapter has highlighted the health concerns associated with physical inactivity. Problems have been identified and a number of encouraging research findings shared. However there is much to be done if the alarming trends of physical inactivity among children and youth are to be reversed. Professor Noakes (2002) in his opening Commonwealth address identified the problems many countries face today. He suggests we must act now and we must be forceful in creating change:

> To influence the global future in a significant meaningful way, we must consider making the promotion of lifelong physical activity one of the most important foci of our profession. To achieve this, we must follow the example of those commercial interests that are our competitors, and exactly as does the fast food industry, ruthlessly and unashamedly target the youth. Instead, by reducing the exposure of children to physical education in schools, we have achieved the exactly opposite effect and, through neglect, have invited the ingress of our more noxious competitors. Since governments are beginning to realize that the prevention of chronic illness is cheaper than its treatment, there is no better time than the present to activate a new, more strident approach to this problem. The guilt of our past failures must be a spur and not a deterrent for renewed action. (p. 10)

Until governments and educational leaders understand the importance of 'mind and body' in their educational decision making, little is likely to change. Physical education must be taken seriously and given the respect it deserves. Only then will children and youth develop the skills, knowledge, and attitudes necessary for the development of healthy active lifestyles. The approach being undertaken in Hong Kong with physical education curriculum reform and teacher in-service and pre-service development is an encouraging start to help combat the inactive lifestyles so common among the young people of today.

References

Berg, S., & Fishburne, G. J. (2002, July). *Health promoting behaviors, lifelong learning and active living: How effectively do teachers use the school physical education curriculum to address these issues?* Paper presented at the Ninth International Literacy & Education Research Network Conference on Learning, Beijing, China.

Chan, K.M., Li, J.X., Hong, Y.L, Leung, S.F. (1998). Health benefits of exercise and diet control in children and adolescents — a Hong Kong and China perspective. In K. M. Chan & L. J. Micheli (Eds.), *Sports and children* (pp. 108-118). Hong Kong: Williams & Wilkins Asia-Pacific.

Curriculum Development Council (1988). Syllabuses for secondary schools physical education (Secondary I–V). Hong Kong: The Government Education Department.

Curriculum Development Council (1995). *Syllabuses for primary schools physical education (Primary 1-6).* Hong Kong: The Government Education Department.

Curriculum Development Council (2002). *Physical education — Key learning area curriculum guide (Primary 1–Secondary 3).* Hong Kong: HKSAR Government Education Department.

Dietz, W. H., & Gortmaker, S. L. (2001). Preventing obesity in children and adolescents. *Annual Review of Public Health, 22,* 337–353.

Eston, R.G., Ingledew, D.K., Fu, F.H., & Rowlands, A. (1998). A Comparison of health-related fitness measures in 7- to15-year olds in Hong Kong and North Wales. In: K. M. Chan & L. J. Micheli (Eds.), *Sports and children* (pp. 119–132). Hong Kong: Williams & Wilkins Asia-Pacific.

Fishburne, G. J. (2002a, July). *Developing and maintaining healthy bones: What children need to learn.* Paper presented at the Ninth International Literacy & Education Research Network Conference on Learning, Beijing, China.

Fishburne, G. J. (2002b, November). *Sensitive times during development: Fundamental movement patterns and physical education.* Invited keynote speach for the Hong Kong Teachers' Conference, The Chinese University of Hong Kong.

Fishburne, G. J., McKay, H., & Berg, S. (2002). Developmentally appropriate activities to improve elementary aged school students' bone development and muscular strength. *Proceedings of the 12th Commonwealth International Sport Conference* (p. 127). London, UK: Commonwealth Universities Publications.

Ha, A. S., Chan, W. K., & Sum, K. M. (2003) *A report on physical education teachers development programme — Conferences and workshops for PE curriculum leaders in primary schools.* Hong Kong: The Chinese University of Hong Kong.

Ha, A. S., Johns, D. P., & Fung, W. M. (2001). Effect of instructional format on appropriate time in motor skills, heart rate intensity and exercise enjoyment of students. *Educational Research Journal, 16,* 239–255.

Ha, A. S., Johns, D. P., & Shiu, E. S. (2003). Students' perspective of the physical education curriculum in Hong Kong. *The Physical Educator, 60*(4), 194–202.

Ha, A. S., Lee, J. C., Chan, W. K., & Sum, R. K. (2004). Teachers' perceptions of in-service teacher training to support curriculum change in physical education: The Hong Kong experience. *Sport, Education, and Society, 9*(3), 421–438.

Ha, A. S., Pang, A. C., & Cheung, K. C. (2004). Perceptions of physical education learning environment of Hong Kong children. *International Journal of Eastern Sports and Physical Education, 2*(1), 49–58.

Ha, A. S., Wong, S. H., Chan, W. K., & Morris, J. (2002). Effects of school-based rope skipping and nutrition programs on Hong Kong school children. *Research Quarterly for Exercise and Sport, 73*(supplement), A68.

Hardman, K., & Marshall, J. J. (2002). *The world-wide survey of the state and status of school physical education.* Manchester, UK: University of Manchester.

Hatano, Y., Hua, Z. D., Jiang, L. D., Fu, F., Zhi, C. J., & Wei, S. D. (1997). Comparative study of physical fitness of the youth in Asia. *Journal of Physical Education & Recreation, 3,* 4–11.

Janus, E. D. (1997). Epidemiology of cardiovascular risk factors in Hong Kong. *Clinical and Experimental Pharmacology and Physiology, 24,* 987–988.

Johns, D. P. & Ha, A. S. (1999). Home and recess physical and dietary behavioral patterns of Hong Kong children. *Research Quarterly for Exercise and Sport, 70:* 3:319–323.

Lindner, K. J. (1998). Sport and activity participation of Hong Kong school children and youth — Part 1. *The Hong Kong Journal of Sports Medicine and Sports Science, 6,*16–27.

Lau, E. M., & Cooper, C. (1993). Epidemiology and prevention of osteoporosis in urbanized Asian populations. *Osteoporosis International, 3* (supplement 1), S23–S26.

Lee, A. S., Critchley, J. A., Chan, J. C., Anderson, P. J., Thomas, G. N., Ko, G. T., Young, R. P., Chan, T. Y., Cockram, C. S., & Tomlinson, B. (2000). Obesity is the key determinant of cardiovascular risk factors in the Hong Kong Chinese population: Cross sectional clinic-based study. *Hong Kong Medical Journal, 6,* 12–23.

Leung, G. M., & Lam, K. S. (2000). Diabetic complications and their implications on health care in Asia. *Hong Kong Medical Journal, 6,* 61–68.

Leung, S. F., Ng, M. Y., & Lau, T. F. (1995). Prevalence of obesity in Hong Kong children and adolescents aged 3-18 years. *Chinese Journal of Preventive Medicine, 19,* 270–272.

Macfarlane, D. J. (1997). *Measuring the habitual physical activity of Hong Kong primary school children: Difficult - disturbing - data.* Symposium on Research in Sports Science and Physical Education. South-East Asia Perspective. The Chinese University of Hong Kong.

Noakes, T. (2002). Quality issues in the exercise sciences. *Proceedings of the 12th Commonwealth International Sport Conference* (pp. 9–13). London: Commonwealth Universities Publications.

Sung, R. Y. T., Yu, C. W., Chang, S. K. Y., Mo, S. W., Woo, K. S., & Lam, C. W. K. (2002). Effects of dietary intervention and strength training on blood lipid level in obese children. *Archives of Diseases in Childhood, 86,* 407–410.

Tremblay, M. S., & Willms, J. D. (2000). Secular trends in the body mass index of Canadian children. *Canadian Medical Association Journal, 163,* 1429–1433.

Woo, J., Leung, S. S., Ho, S. C., Sham, A., Lam, T. H., & Janus, E. D. (1999). Influence of educational level marital status on dietary intake, obesity and other cardiovascular risk factors in a Hong Kong Chinese population. *European Journal of Clinical Nutrition, 53,* 461–467.

CHAPTER 14

The Future of School Physical Education in Perspective

Koenraad J. Lindner

Macfarlane concluded in Chapter 4 of this book that children in Hong Kong must be among the least physically active in the world. Anecdotal evidence, along with the scientific data presented in several other chapters (McManus, Chapter 5; Sit, Chow, & Lindner, Chapter 6), appears to support such a view. Take a look at the inside area of the Happy Valley racecourse in early mornings: a good number of people exercising, but they are all adults and mostly elderly. On Sundays the pitches there are heavily used, but again by adults and almost exclusively men, the exception being an organized practice for rugby club boys and a few girls. On weekday afternoons there is no child to be found other than those in school uniform on their way home and a few preschoolers playing on the monkey bars guarded by their maids. Pass by a playground in the city and you will see men playing soccer and basketball and occasionally volleyball. Where are the kids?

Sadly, there seems to be no time or space for children to play active games. In the morning they need to be dragged out of bed, still exhausted from homework, TV watching and late-night dinner. In the afternoon they are facing a new mountain of homework, and they would have to compete with adolescents and adults for facilities if there were an opportunity to go out and play. In the weekends, family dinners, visits, shopping trips, church or temple attendance and of course homework will leave little time for recreation of a physical nature. The lucky ones will occasionally be taken on a walk or hike with their family.

We silence our conscience by arguing that physical activity is provided by the school, in the PE lessons. We only realize how false this self-assurance is when we learn that the energy expended in the typical PE class is next to nothing (Chapter 4, Macfarlane, and Chapter 13, Ha & Fishburne). The kids do more physical work walking up and down the stairs to go to their academic classes than in the gym, or the school's puny playground that doubles as 'gymnasium'. They hardly ever break a sweat, which at 28 degrees Celsius and 90 percent humidity should be so easy to accomplish. Granted, a number of school children will participate in after-school intramural sports or inter school leagues and derive some physical activity from practices and competitions, but this tends to be ad-hoc, for a few and at low levels, particularly so for the girls. There is an overemphasis on team sports in those programmes while there is little room for other forms of physical activity such as dance and aerobics. There are also kids who engage in serious training in sport clubs, but this is expensive and requires parents or maids to take them, and therefore is only feasible for the well-to-do. There is no evidence supporting a claim that the school succeeds in providing for the physical activity a growing child needs for optimal development.

With insufficient exercise in the school and virtually none outside of school, Hong Kong children are frightfully sedentary. They are destined to become uncoordinated, unfit, overweight, illness-prone adults. It is high time to address the question: what are we going to do about it? While the problem is clear and the consequences obvious as outlined in this volume (chapters by Thomas et al., Sung et al.), arriving at solutions will be extremely difficult.

Physical Activity: Where and When?

Hong Kong children need to be a lot more physically active; this is generally agreed. Both where and when are problematic questions. Jim Dickinsen discussed a range of possibilities for increasing facilities and opportunities for physical activity in Chapter 12. If we are serious in our efforts to get our children to engage more in physical activities, we must allocate the necessary resources for improving and expanding the facilities to make this possible. However, there is no point in spending on facilities if there is not going to be an increase in sport and exercise participation. As argued above, a large component of the cause of low participation in physical activities is that many kids have little time to engage in them. The average Hong Kong school kid is grossly overloaded with academic homework, the importance and benefits of which are in turn grossly overestimated by teachers and parents. Schools would serve the interest of students a lot better if a proportion of 'homework' were to consist of physical activities!

Of course homework is not the only impediment to a healthy dose of habitual physical exercise. Hong Kong children, as are their parents, are an inactive (some say 'lazy') bunch, so conditioned by culture, tradition, climate and living conditions (Chapter 11, Johns & Vertinsky, and Chapter 12, Dickinson). Passive recreation, especially TV watching and computering, are massively preferred above anything that involves the expenditure of even moderate amounts of energy. If we don't re-educate our population, we can have the best and the most facilities in the world and create ample time for sport and exercise, but there will still be no change in participation. Hong Kong people need to be taught to appreciate the importance and the joy of being physically active. This is best done when the learner is young and impressionable. So, as Au (Chapter 9), Johns (Chapter 10) and Ha and Fishburne (Chapter 13) surmised, the key to the solution lies in the school, and therefore with school physical education. The problem is that school PE does not seem to be designed to accomplish this, or at least has not succeeded in bringing this attitude about.

School Physical Education: Who and What?

There is no doubt that the PE lessons in schools need to be drastically changed. They don't appear to serve any purpose at this time other than perhaps to provide a short respite from the drudgery of the academic subjects. Even as a diversion PE is disliked by many; a sure sign it is not recognized as something desirable or important, even by the students! It is easy to say change is needed, but it is a different thing to determine the what and the who of it. The crux of the matter is indeed the who and the what, two components of a powerful inertial force that resists change and progress. Who is going to modernize the PE curriculum and the way it is taught? There is little hope this will come from the serving PE teachers, who have a strong tendency to teach the way they were taught, the way they were taught to teach, and the way they have always been teaching. Given their limited professional training, heavy teaching loads, marginalisation of their subject and widespread low morale, an impetus from that direction cannot realistically be expected. Many Hong Kong PE teachers perform miracles given their working conditions and expectations, and, as Cecilia Au describes in Chapter 9, they are the most frequently mentioned agent to encourage students to engage in physical activity. But they are unlikely to emerge as agents of change. Similar low expectations apply to the teacher-trainers, who either are under-qualified to teach change, or will be bogged down in their theoretical debates about what is needed and why. Their vested interests are unlikely to be set aside in favour of radical changes they do not understand, accept or wish to be bothered with.

It is expected that a complete overhaul of the PE curriculum and teaching approach would require at least a generation; more likely half a century. Even if by some miracles we could agree on the what and how today and receive the necessary political cooperation for their implementation tomorrow, it would take years of re-tooling teacher-trainers, four more years to instruct student-teachers in the what and the how, and a decade or more to phase out the teachers who are not on track and to begin seeing the benefits in the change. With such a seemingly insurmountable task ahead, wouldn't it be better to leave things the way they are and just try to improve here and there? This would certainly be more convenient, less costly, quicker and less controversial, but still the answer is NO. We cannot afford to muddle on in the blind hope that things will improve. There is too much at stake. It is clear that the current approach is no longer suitable for this changing society, and stopgap measures will not be sufficient. The present lack of physical activity (Chapters, 4, 5 and 6) and the deleterious consequences thereof in our youngsters (Chapters 7 and 8) have been documented in this book and many other publications, and it is time to act and adopt an approach that is capable of instilling in our citizens the notion that physical activity is as necessary for modern life as food, sleep, practical skills and knowledge.

That brings us to the question: What should be taught in the PE lesson? Looking back in history we learn the approaches that have *not* been successful (even though we are still clinging to their retention in today's curriculum). The aims of physical education have varied considerably since Turnvater Jahn. An early purpose was to prepare physically able men for warfare through marching, calisthenics and gymnastics. The term 'physical training' is still in use here and there, but the objective of producing able cannon fodder is no longer fashionable. Another goal of physical education once was "character formation" through engagement in competitive sport, which also had a useful physical component that cynics would say was indistinguishable from the cannon fodder philosophy. However, a more positive formulation of the desired outcomes included fitness, skill, strategy and fair play. When American politicians were advised how embarrassingly unfit children were in comparison to those on the other side of the Atlantic, the fitness-focus disaster commenced. If kids are unfit, the reasoning went, they should be made fit. The PE class activities changed into sit-ups, jumping jacks and bent-arm hangs, the scores on the fitness tests improved dramatically (miracle of miracles!), and the approach was declared a grand success. Until it became clear that (a) the kids were still poor on any items not included in the fitness test batteries, (b) they hated PE classes and swore never to do another push-up in their life, and (c) many never attained the criteria set for 'success' and resigned themselves to hopelessness and inactivity.

Then another go at sports, mostly established competitive sports, but this time with different aims: prepare for participation at advanced levels and for continued involvement in the adult years. The "competence motivation" hypothesis lent credence to this approach. It postulates that children are in sport to savour the satisfaction of mastering skills and realizing their potentials. The achievements in turn would motivate continued participation after the school years. The PE lessons would be the first training grounds for future professionals and olympians! With the knowledge and skills of the games the appreciative recipients would engage in life-long participation! Lofty goals, but utterly delusory. It works reasonable well for the few athletically inclined and motorically gifted, but most others tune out, feel inadequate, are turned off, disengage, and very few, even among the 'stars', continue participation beyond the school years. And we still force-feed soccer and basketball to those not hungry for them, and we still teach the shot put in the hope that the learners will continue this activity until their eighties. Are we intellectually challenged, or are we so steeped in tradition that we have lost the ability or will to search for other avenues?

Whereto From Here?

It is easy to speculate on where change will not be coming from, and to lampoon past approaches that are found to have been faulty. Where have we gone wrong in our thinking? I believe the current PE approach has been spectacularly unsuccessful because it followed two erroneous assumptions. The first is the belief that we can actually impart proficiency in sport skills and/or make the children fit in the PE lessons. It is time to face the truth, however painful: this is impossible. Both are products of lifestyle commitments and can't be accomplished through a meagre hour of PE lessons per week. Trying to accomplish them anyway will have negative consequences, as the futility of it will demoralize both teachers and students. Defenders of the current system will argue that the PE lesson lays the foundation for sport skills and fitness, to be perfected outside of school. The reality is, as argued earlier, there *is* no outside of school involvement for most kids either by choice or by circumstance, and the PE lesson comprises the extent of their weekly physical activity. For them it is like trying to learn piano playing in weekly sessions without access to the instrument in between lessons: it will never get anywhere. Again, the approach may suit a few students who are involved in sport clubs after school or who pursue personal fitness goals, but the majority will find the class activities uninteresting, useless and a prolific source of perceived failures. In fact, progressing interested students will soon find the activities too elementary and feel frustrated by the low performance level of the class so that they become bored and annoyed also. 'Acquiring sport skills' and 'attaining fitness' should *not* be objectives of school physical education, simply because they are unattainable.

The other main faulty assumption has been the belief that we can teach PE to a class of youngsters and treat them as a homogeneous group (perhaps this is the mistake of school education in general!). Think about it: it is akin to sending them to a physician for group diagnosis and a collective prescription to be dispensed in equal doses to all. A few may be helped, but most will get sicker. But it is cheap and convenient. I am not presenting this as a novel idea. Maria Montessori based her education system on the same notion a century ago. It turned out the individual approach worked brilliantly for the gifted and self-motivated, not so well for the mediocre and disinterested students. An historical lesson is to be learned from this as well, as in principle the Montessori method is sound, but it suffered in its effectiveness because of inadequate implementation.

So, PE should *not* be taught with the traditional group approach method and should *not* have the objectives we have long thought to be essential. What then is physical education and how should it be taught? The answers flow from a reconsideration of the purpose of physical education. In my mind, a physically educated person is one who:

- is aware of and accepts the necessity of physical activity for attaining and maintaining well-being,
- has the desire to keep the body functioning optimally and to combat decline associated with disease and aging, and
- has the knowledge and skills to adequately self-prescribe, self-monitor and self-evaluate the level of physical activity in relation to the state of the body, and knows where to turn for help when required.

In other words, the purpose of physical education is to teach people how to take responsibility for their own physical wellness.

Note that the above statement of purposes does not include the objective of making the individual *like* physical activity. Such aim is ludicrous since people would select activities they like, or ones they dislike least, or ones they perceive they need whether they like them or not. As with skill and fitness, 'liking' is a serendipitous outcome, but an unattainable goal. By the same token, it is counterproductive to specify what skills and activities must be included in a curriculum, because this would imply that these will be forced upon all students whether receptive to them or not. Frequently claimed social and moral benefits of sport and exercise participation are also inappropriate as objectives. They may well be welcome occasional by-products, but can never be attained as designated goals of physical education as defined here. Similarly, I am not excluding athletic brilliance as a desirable outcome, but it should never be an explicit objective of PE.

The Ensuing School PE Curriculum

Would such a drastic reformulation of PE's objectives not have far-reaching consequences for school physical education? The answer is 'yes' in some respects, and 'no' in other. The main change would be in how PE would be 'taught', especially at the secondary school level. We would not need more gymnasiums or other sport facilities than is currently standard for schools (although access to outdoor facilities will be an enviable commodity), and we would not need more hours of physical education classes on the time table. We would not need more PE teachers, but instead ones that are differently trained. The students would not normally play soccer and basketball or collectively practise track and field techniques during the PE lesson, but rather work on their personal objectives with the PE teacher as a consultant. There would be no performance tests with absolute standards to determine grades or other evaluations, and no student would be compared to any other student about anything. There would be no need to separate the genders for the PE lessons, and there would be no formal competition among the students during the lessons.

Apart from the changes in the nature of the physical education lesson, there will have to be major adjustments in the child's environment outside of school. Since physical activity 'quota' cannot possibly be met during the PE lessons, the child must exercise in some form before or after school. First, the family members must accommodate this by permitting, no, encouraging and facilitating the child to be physically active, and join in where possible. Acceptance is needed of (self-)assigned physical activity 'homework' as natural and desirable. Second, the school must adjust to the new system and make room for PE 'homework' by reducing out-of-class assignments in the other subjects to more reasonable levels, thus assuring that the students will have time to exercise both brain and body. They must continue to provide opportunities for participation in recreational or competitive sport for those who prefer these forms of physical activity. Third, youth sport clubs also have an important role to play in this system and need to be strongly supported by community and government. Fourth, the authorities must make sure that there are sufficient and adequate facilities for children and youth to make fulfilling the commitments to their wellness programme possible. Finally, rather substantial changes would be required in the education of the PE teacher. In addition to being qualified to teach basic and sport-like activities, he or she would need thorough training in physical activity prescription, monitoring and evaluation as well as in consultancy-related knowledges and skills. All aspects of PE teacher training should fit with the revised statement of purpose.

This is not the place to present a detailed school PE curriculum and the above are some thoughts immediately emanating from the re-conceptualization of PE's purpose. It would take time and thorough consideration to translate the concept into a complete system of PE delivery, and probably years until society will be ready to endorse and implement it. Nevertheless, here are some initial basic principles that come to mind for a 'responsibility for our own physical wellness' approach to school physical education.

(1) Progressive transition from enjoyment focus to responsibility-for-own-wellness focus.
(2) Progressive transition from group learning and doing to individual learning and doing.
(3) Progressive transition from teacher-selected to student-selected physical activities.
(4) Progressive change from a prescribing PE teacher to an advising and monitoring PE teacher.
(5) Instilling in the student, as early as possible, the notion of their responsibility for their own level of physical activity.
(6) Progressively increasing the knowledge component of the

PE lesson, both in terms of time spent and as basis for evaluation.

(7) Progress in attaining appropriate personal goals as partial basis for evaluation in secondary school.

The challenge that lies ahead is to make the relevant parties acknowledge that changes in school PE are needed and to assure adoption of the concept presented here. A new curriculum based on the changed view of physical education's purpose needs to be developed along with proposals for changes in PE teacher training. Monumental tasks, but ones we should start today rather than tomorrow. It is no exaggeration to state that the health of the nation is at stake.

It is satisfying to note from Ha and Fishburne's Chaper 13, that a change in approach to the PE curriculum has begun in Hong Kong, very much in line with the reasoning presented here. It seems fair to speculate that the contributions of the researchers in the area of physical activity and health-related behaviour (many of them authors of chapters in this book) have been instrumental in exposing the seriousness of the current problem and its consequences and in stimulating implementation of the much needed change.

Contributing Authors

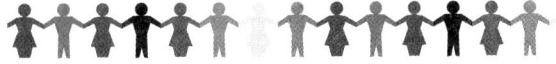

Cecilia Au, The University of Hong Kong

Before joining HKU in 1994, Ms Au lectured at the Grantham and Sir Robert Black Colleges of Education, and served as head of Physical Education for the five Technical Institutes at the Vocational Training Council, and as an Inspector of Schools for the Hong Kong Government's Advisory Inspectorate. She has served as Coordinator of Physical Education and Student Sports Programmes at the Institute of Human Performance of the Hong Kong University and has been Manager of Promotion and Marketing and the Institute's liaison with the student union's Sports Association. Her main academic interests are the study of the motivational profiles of athletes in the framework of reversal theory, socialization in sports participation, and gender issues. She holds a B.A. from the University of Auckland and a M.Sc. from Leicester University. From 2003–05, Ms Au was a member of the Women & Sport Commission, Sports Federation & Olympic Committee of Hong Kong, China.

Norman Chan, The Chinese University of Hong Kong

Norman Chan is currently Honorary Associate Professor in the Department of Medicine & Therapeutics. He is also the Clinical Director at the Qualigenics Diabetes Centre. He completed his MD thesis in "Endothelial dysfunction in Diabetes" at University College London, UK in 2002. His research interests include endothelial dysfunction and insulin resistance. He is an author of over 60 publications and several book chapters. He is also a regular speaker at national and international meetings.

Ken Chow, Canossa Primary School, Hong Kong

Mr Chow Chi Kin obtained his Ph.D. from the University of Hong Kong in 2003 with research in children and youth's sport participation. He has served as a part-time Lecturer/Tutor at The University of Hong Kong, The Hong Kong Baptist University and the Open University of Hong Kong over the past several years. He was a Minute Secretary of the Hong Kong Physical Education Teachers Society in 2000. Ken has served as a Teacher Development Consultant at the Hong Kong Institute of Education (HKIEd) with major areas of work on developing mentoring and peer review skills. In addition to the study of the bio-psycho-social aspects and the social-cognitive models of youth sport participation, pedagogical content knowledge and curriculum of physical education are the current research interests of Dr Chow who serves at present as a principal of a primary school.

Clive Cockram, The Chinese University of Hong Kong

Clive Cockram is a Professor of Medicine in the Department of Medicine and Therapeutics. He took up this teaching position, initially as a Senior Lecturer, in Hong Kong in 1985 having completed his undergraduate and post-graduate trainings at St Thomas' Hospital Medical School, University of London and at St George's Hospital, London respectively. He returned to St Thomas' Hospital, where he was the holder of a MRC Research Training Fellowship and later a lectureship in the Department of Medicine. He set up the Division of Endocrinology and Diabetes in the Department in Hong Kong and is now assisting also with the development of an Infectious Diseases Division. His main research interest is Type 2 diabetes mellitus. He has published more than 300 papers, articles and book chapters. He has also been extensively involved in the activities of the International Diabetes Federation both in the Western Pacific Region and at the global level.

Jim Dickinson, University of Calgary

James A Dickinson MBBS (Queensland) PhD (Newcastle) FRACGP, FAFPHM, CCFP (Can) is Professor of Family Medicine at the University of Calgary. He was formerly Professor of Family Medicine in the Department of Community and Family Medicine at The Chinese

University of Hong Kong (1997–2002), and at the University of Western Australia (1994–1997). He was Consulting Adviser in General Practice to the Department of Health in Canberra (1990–1994). He has a special interest in researching preventive activities such as the screening for disease, behaviour change of doctors, their patients and the populations from which they come. His research spans from clinical and epidemiological to educational and sociological. He regarded his time in Hong Kong as being a five years participant-observational research in adapting ideas and methods from Western society to a developing blend of old and new China in Hong Kong.

Graham Fishburne, University of Alberta

Graham received his formal education in England and Canada. He holds a B.Sc. degree (Newcastle) in electrical and electronic engineering and is a qualified professional engineer (P.Eng.) before embarking on a teaching career. He received his teacher education at the Loughborough University and taught at both the elementary and secondary levels before entering graduate school. He obtained a masters degree in education (Manchester) and a doctoral degree (Alberta) before completing a post-doctoral fellowship in the Department of Psychology at the University of Alberta. He currently is Professor of Education and Associate Director of the Institute for Olympic Education at the University of Alberta in Canada. He has received numerous research and teaching awards for his university work. He has published over 100 research articles and one of his textbooks on elementary school physical education is used as a standard course text in over 200 universities and colleges in the US and Canada.

Amy Ha, The Chinese University of Hong Kong

Amy Ha obtained her first degree in physical education from Fu Jen Catholic University in Taiwan and her master and doctoral degrees in sport pedagogy at Springfield College and Walden University respectively in United States. She is currently Professor in the Department of Sports Science and Physical Education and Associate Director of the Centre for University and School Partnership at The Chinese University of Hong Kong. Her research areas included critical pedagogy, teacher development and teaching effectiveness. Over the past five years she has received a substantial research grant and has published her research results in both local and international academic journals extensively. She is also the founder and President of the Hong Kong Rope Skipping Association.

Stanley Hui, The Chinese University of Hong Kong

Stanley Sai-chuen Hui is an Associate Professor in the Department of Sports Science and Physical Education, a fellow of the American College of Sports Medicine (ACSM), and a fellow of the American Alliance for Health, Physical Education, Recreation and Dance. A physical education teacher since 1985, he received a B.P.E. (1991) and an M.Sc. degree in Health and Fitness (1992) at Springfield College, and a doctoral degree in Exercise Science from the University of Houston. Dr. Hui has been certified as a Health Fitness Director by the ACSM in 2000, and is serving as the Certification Director of the ACSM Health Fitness Instructor Examination in Hong Kong. He is also a vice-chairman of the Physical Fitness Association of Hong Kong. Dr Hui's specialization is in measurement research in physical fitness and health. Besides teaching and research at the university, he spends most of his time promoting correct concepts of active lifestyle and health.

David Johns, The Chinese University of Hong Kong

David Johns is Reader and Chairman of the Department of Sports Science and Physical Education at The Chinese University of Hong Kong. After receiving his teacher training at Exeter University he moved to Canada and attended the University of Alberta where he received his PhD in Physical education in 1979. Served in a wide range of teaching positions at all levels of education and for the last 30 years has taught at universities in the United Kingdom, Canada, Australia and Hong Kong. Previously a Professor of Physical Education, at the University of Manitoba, Winnipeg, Canada he was named Assistant Olympic Coach to the 1976 Canadian Men's Gymnastic Team and was a sport consultant to athletes on international teams in a wide range of Olympic sports. Research interests in Hong Kong have focused on school curriculum policy and practice, and the sociological and ecological factors that influence physical activity and health practices.

Koenraad Lindner, The University of Hong Kong

After obtaining his teacher qualifications from the Academy of Physical Education in The Hague, The Netherlands, Koenraad pursued graduate studies in Toledo, Ohio, USA, earning M.Ed. and Ph.D. degrees. He taught and conducted research at the University of Manitoba, Canada for 18 years before moving to Hong Kong in 1992. He retired in 2001 from the post of Department Head of the Physical Education and Sports Science Unit, now the Institute of Human Performance of the University of Hong Kong. His research areas included aspects of motor learning and control, epidemiology of sports injuries, sport participation and withdrawal, and the motivational aspects of physical activity participation. His publication record comprises some 85 books, book chapters and articles.

Duncan Macfarlane, The University of Hong Kong

Duncan is an Associate Professor and Assistant Director of the Institute of Human Performance, having previously been a Lecturer in the School of Physical Education, University of Otago, New Zealand. His qualifications include BPhEd (Otago), BSc(Hons: First Class: Otago), D.Phil. (Oxford) and he is an accredited Level 3 exercise physiologist (SSNZ) and anthropometrist (ISAK). His teaching and research covers a variety of courses in human stress physiology and he has published over 30 refereed articles; 14 chapters/reports; 40 conference/academic presentations and has supervised 80 undergraduates and postgraduate dissertations. He currently researches levels of habitual physical activity in young children and the elderly, the control of ventilation, and the measurement of exercise performance.

Ali McManus, The University of Hong Kong

Ali McManus joined the University of Hong Kong in 1994 from the University of Exeter, where she graduated with a First Class honours degree in 1990 and a PhD in 1994 under the supervision of Professor Neil Armstrong. Her primary research interest lies in the under-standing of children's exercise and physical activity responses in health and disease. Interest in the plasticity of both cardiopulmonary function and physical activity has been expanded to explore the effect of different types of exercise stimuli on cardiopulmonary function, as well as innovative ways to increase physical activity.

Tony Nelson, The Chinese University of Hong Kong

Tony Nelson is a Professor in Paediatrics at The Chinese University of Hong Kong. He studied medicine at the University of Cape Town in South Africa and received a Doctor of Medicine degree from the University of Otago, New Zealand. Dr Nelson has worked in various regions around the world, including the Middle East, Africa and Asia. Since arriving in Hong Kong from 1993, his research has focused on sudden infant death syndrome, child care practices, diarrhoea, breastfeeding and obesity.

Cindy Sit, The University of Hong Kong

Cindy Sit is a Research Assistant Professor in the Institute of Human Performance (IHP) of The University of Hong Kong, where she earned both M.Phil. and Ph.D. degrees. She joined the IHP in February 2004 from the Department of Physical Education and Sports Science, The Hong Kong Institute of Education. Her research interests include sport participation patterns and motivation in children with and without disabilities, motivational orientations and profiles of children and youth, and adapted physical activity. She is currently an Executive Board Member on Asian Society of Adapted Physical Education and Exercise (ASAPE) representing China.

Raymond Sum, The Chinese University of Hong Kong

Raymond Sum is a physical education instructor at The Chinese University of Hong Kong. He studied physical education at the National Taiwan Normal University in Taipei and completed his Master of Physical Education in Springfield College, U.S.A. He served as an executive committee member in promoting health and fitness in the Physical Fitness Association of Hong Kong. He is also the author of a well-known Chinese fitness theory book entitled *Foundation of Physical Fitness* published by the Physical Fitness Association of Hong Kong. He is appointed lecturer, examiner and workshop coordinator of the health fitness instructor certification of the American College of Sports Medicine after obtaining his professional health fitness instructor certification in 1998.

Rita Sung, The Chinese University of Hong Kong
Rita Sung is a professor at the Department of Paediatrics, The Chinese University of Hong Kong. She studied medicine at the National Taiwan University in Taipei and received a Doctor of Medicine degree from the University of Wales, Cardiff. She is a fellow of the Royal College of Paediatrics and Child Health UK. Her subspecialty is paediatric cardiology. Her research interest is on cardiopulmonary function and preventive cardiology.

G. Neil Thomas, The University of Hong Kong
Neil Thomas is an Assistant Professor in the Department of Community Medicine. He completed his M.Phil. in the Department of Microbiology of The Chinese University of Hong Kong in viral molecular epidemiology, and later his Ph.D. in genetic epidemiology of hypertension and associated conditions including obesity in the Department of Medicine and Therapeutics at the same university. His research interests include the pathogenesis of the metabolic syndrome for which obesity is a major underlying risk factor. He is an author of over 90 publications, over 60 of which are with indexed journals. He has given invited lectures on obesity and the metabolic syndrome both locally and internationally.

Brian Tomlinson, The Chinese University of Hong Kong
Brian Tomlinson is Professor and Head of the Division of Clinical Pharmacology in the Department of Medicine and Therapeutics at The Chinese University of Hong Kong. He graduated from the Middlesex Hospital Medical School, University of London and completed training in internal medicine in Dundee and then at The University College Hospital, London where he specialised in Clinical Pharmacology and completed his MD. He joined The Chinese University of Hong Kong in 1990. His research interests include the pathogenesis and treatment of hyperlipidaemia, hypertension and the metabolic syndrome, and the clinical pharmacology of cardiovascular drugs and herbal medicines. He is an author of over 200 publications and over 350 abstracts and has given numerous invited lectures.

Patricia Vertinsky, University of British Columbia

Patricia Vertinsky is Professor of Human Kinetics and a Distinguished University Scholar at UBC. Her research program focuses upon the history of the gendered body, especially in relation to health and physical activity. She is a Fellow of the Academy of Kinesiology and Physical Education, a former President of the North American Society of Sport History, and Vice-President of the International Society for Physical Education and Sport History. She has authored and edited a number of books and articles, including *The Eternally Wounded Woman: Doctors and Exercise in the Late 19th Century; Sites of Sport; Space, Place and Experience* (with John Bale) and *Memory, Monument and Modernism: Disciplining the Body in the Gymnasium* (with Sherry Mckay). Her current project is focused on Dartington Hall and a remarkable series of 'educators of the body' who passed through there during the 1930's. She is also co-editing a book on *Physical Culture, Power and the Body* with Jennifer Hargreaves.

Stephen Wong, The Chinese University of Hong Kong

Stephen Wong is a Professor at the Department of Sports Science and Physical Education, The Chinese University of Hong Kong. He earned his M.Sc. and Ph.D. degrees in exercise physiology at Loughborough University. His overseas experience combined with the local knowledge of Hong Kong schools has enabled him to introduce a successful early morning exercise programme to primary schools in Hong Kong. His research interests, all associated with energy systems of the body, explore the use of the glycemic index in determining the choice of pre-competition foods and the issues of hydration during exercise in hot environments. He is also a Fellow of the American College of Sports Medicine.